The **7** MINUTE BACK PAIN SOLUTION

The

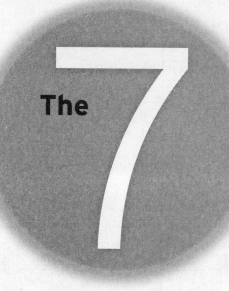

7

MINUTE
BACK PAIN
SOLUTION

7 Simple Exercises
to Heal Your Back in Just Minutes a Day

GERARD GIRASOLE, M.D. AND CARA HARTMAN, CPT

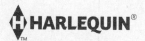

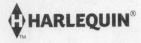

THE 7-MINUTE BACK PAIN SOLUTION

ISBN-13: 978-0-373-89258-7

Photographs by Scott Wynn

Line drawings by Victoria Skomal Wilchinsky

The ideas, procedures and suggestions contained in this book are not intended as a substitute for consulting with your physician. All matters regarding your health require medical supervision.

Library of Congress Cataloging-in-Publication Data

Girasole, Gerard.

   The 7-minute back pain solution / by Gerard Girasole and Cara Hartman ; with Karen Moline.

      p. cm.

   Includes index.

   ISBN 978-0-373-89258-7

   1. Backache--Exercise therapy. 2. Back exercises. I. Hartman, Cara. II. Moline, Karen. III. Title. IV. Title: Seven minute back pain solution.

   RD768.G57 2012

   617.5´64062--dc23

                        2011028259

www.Harlequin.com

Printed in U.S.A.

CONTENTS

INTRODUCTION

COMEDIANS USED TO JOKE about headaches when they said, "Not tonight, honey." But they got it wrong. Back pain is the real passion killer.

Dealing with this pain is not just about personal suffering—it's an enormous issue with grave implications for the economics of the workplace and our struggling health-care system. The statistics are telling: at least 80 percent of all adults suffer from a bout of lower back pain at some point in their lifetime, with over thirty-one million Americans in pain from backaches at any given time, and nearly one-quarter of all American adults experiencing at least one day of back pain every three months.

Because you use your back in so much of what you do, and because back pain is often so debilitating, it is second only to the common cold as a cause of lost time from work, and it causes more loss of productivity in the workplace than any other medical condition—to the tune of fifty billion dollars in losses each year just in the United States. According to "Understanding Pain," the cover story of the March 7, 2011, issue of *Time* magazine, lower back pain accounts for ninety-three million workdays lost every year. It consumes over five billion dollars in health-care costs.

Yet for such a common and chronic problem, the treatment and management of back pain is often rife with misinformation—which can lead to inappropriate treatments. I can say that because as an orthopedic surgeon specializing in spines, I hear it firsthand from my patients.

I know how they feel because I am a back pain sufferer myself. Back pain is an occupational hazard for surgeons, who bend over patients for hours on end in the operating theater.

So I can empathize with how back pain can make you feel as if you are a prisoner in your own body. It can ruin your life, your marriage, your ability to concentrate at work and even your recreation time with your family (try going on the rides at Disney World when you can't walk without wincing!). It can make you too frightened to drive (what if your back seizes up and it's agony to move your foot off the gas pedal?), too worried to have sex (what if you get stuck in a compromising position while in the throes of passion?) and even too embarrassed to get down on your knees to pray in your house of worship (what if it hurts too much to get up again?).

This pain can be compounded by the skeptical or cruel comments made about the amount of pain you're in. Back pain isn't a visible wound. But just because your boss or loved ones can't see it doesn't mean it isn't there.

The patients who come to me all have one thing in common: they are very frightened that their pain means they have a permanently debilitating and serious injury, and that they will be living with pain for life. I know that many of these patients had put off seeing a medical professional because either they couldn't afford a series of visits in our current economy or they automatically assumed they would need surgery and were too afraid to get to the root of their problem. So they self-medicated or tried all sorts of treatments that, over time, only made things worse. Had they come to a spine specialist first, they might have gotten at least some instant psychological relief as they would have been told what you're going to learn in this book, which is that most people with lower back pain do not need surgery or even physical therapy in order to get better and live pain-free lives.

I explain to these patients that sometimes there is absolutely no way to know that their back is about to start throbbing, so they should stop blaming themselves for the situation. The pain can come on when you hit a golf ball the wrong way, pick up your fussing toddler or bend over to tie a shoelace. It can come on when you are sitting at your desk, watching TV or having a slow stroll down the street after dinner.

Other times, back pain starts due to a muscle imbalance. Perhaps your abdominal muscles are stronger than your opposing back muscles, and over time the back muscles just can't handle the stresses put on them. Or these muscles may be strong, but you twist or turn or bend over the wrong way when you're hurrying through the airport or lifting a weight that is too heavy at the gym.

Back pain can also occur because you exercise too little or too much. Or your posture at work might be the culprit. It's hard to remember to sit tall when your workstation is all wrong for your height, but if you sit hunched over at your desk for long periods, your muscles will invariably tense and tighten.

When you're in pain, though, all you want to do is get out of it. This book will make the fear of back pain and the panic disappear, as it will tell you what to do, why you're doing it and how to move precisely *in that moment* and *for that particular situation*—no matter where you are and what you're doing, and no matter how mundane the task at hand. Armed with this knowledge, you will be able to move and to manage the situation. You will no longer experience panic, which can be as debilitating as the pain itself.

Even better, this book will not only bust the myths about back pain but give you a foolproof, daily system for strengthening your back so that bouts of back pain are much less likely to recur.

HOW THE 7-MINUTE BACK PAIN SOLUTION CAME TO BE

I've lost track of how many patients over the years have begged me for a "take-home program" they could easily follow. They often went for professional treatments (chiropractic, physical therapy) and got temporary relief, but they couldn't continue to get great results at home, when they needed them most. This is incredibly frustrating to me and to my colleagues. Our patients suffer and spend a lot of money to get better—while being forced to take time off from work and from their daily lives—yet once they start to heal, they have no idea what to do to maintain or strengthen their backs.

I was thinking about how to solve this dilemma about seven years ago, when a patient named Cara Hartman told me about a sneeze.

Twenty years ago, shortly after the birth of her son, all it took was one sneeze for Cara's back to go into spasms. (Yes, sneezing and coughing can be triggers for pain, just as shoveling snow or playing too much golf on a sunny day can be triggers.) The pain was so unbearable—worse, she told me, than her drug-free childbirth—that she was shocked when the physician in the ER told her she had "only" sprained her lower back. After a month of taking potent prescription painkillers and living in fear that she would never be pain free, she slowly got better. However, the pain suddenly returned several months later, this time radiating down from her right buttock to behind her knee. She couldn't stand up straight, her hips were visibly uneven and it hurt just to breathe. Her local orthopedic surgeon looked at her X-rays and MRI, then told her that she had degenerative disc disease and that if it worsened, she might need surgery to fuse her vertebrae together to lessen the pain and degeneration.

Declining such a radical step, Cara barely managed to cope; the pain was so fierce, she couldn't bear to be touched, which put a tremendous strain on her marriage. She joked to me that she frequented chiropractors as if they were hairdressers, but while their manipulations gave her some relief, her chiropractors offered no preventative measures, such as stretches or exercises she could do on her own once she left their offices.

After an episode of pain so severe it left her stranded on her bedroom floor for two hours, she came to see me. When I viewed her MRI, I saw several degenerative, bulging discs. I was able to allay her fears by telling her that many people suffer from these issues, and that proper therapy might alleviate the pain.

After a number of treatments (physiotherapy, chiropractic therapy, low-dose steroids and heat), which stopped working after several months, Cara came back, and I told her to start doing exercises for her core, as well as stretching the hamstring muscles at the back of her thighs. She laughed and told me I was nuts, because she couldn't believe that simple leg stretches could do anything when she felt as if a knife was running down her back.

I didn't see Cara again for five years, until I ran into her at our local gym. She was amazingly fit and moved with grace and strength, unlike the patient she'd once been. When I complimented her, she told me she'd become so determined to manage her back pain—and to keep exercising and getting stronger—that she'd become a certified personal trainer. Her new profession had enabled her not only to manage her own back pain but to help others move and exercise when they had pain, too.

"First I started stretching my muscles. Then I started working on strengthening my core, and finally I incorporated everything I'd learned from all the years of physical therapy I had," she told me. "It had been so difficult for me because every physical therapist I saw had me do something different. There was no one standardized treatment plan that worked no matter where the pain was. So I was never able to remember anything they told me, and I got really frustrated, until I started asking questions and taking notes. I combined everything I was told with the training I was doing to become certified, and I eventually created my own treatment and recovery plan. With *my* plan, I have had a lot less pain, it hasn't been as intense, and it doesn't last as long." Then she smiled. "Besides, why rely on someone else to fix you if you can do it yourself?"

I have to admit I was extremely impressed, joking that she was trying to put me out of business even as I confessed that my own back was bothering me. Then I watched as she began stretching and training one of my former patients, who'd had spinal fusion surgery. After only a few minutes I couldn't stand it any longer and joined the workout session. When we were done, I was amazed. My back felt strong, and I was able to bend naturally without any pain.

I knew that Cara was on to something unique. She had literally healed her back pain through her self-devised, super-short program of stretches and core routines. We decided to join forces to combine the best of our knowledge as back-pain sufferers and as professionals. We coupled my surgical skills, and my deep understanding of how and why back pain occurs and how best to treat it, with Cara's back-pain prevention tips for daily living and her exacting skills as a personal trainer who knows how best to strengthen and stretch the muscles that support your back and how to ease your aching back. Not only is Cara a personal trainer, but she is someone who has lived with back pain for over twenty years and can certainly empathize with anyone in pain.

Throughout my professional career, I have always been amazed by the lack of knowledge that my patients and the average person have about what causes low back pain and what they can do to treat it. I see thousands of patients each year who come to me specifically for low back pain, and I spend my days in the office explaining how their spine and muscles work, trying to give them an effective visualization of why they're in pain.

While back-pain treatment has seen many advances in regard to surgery, medical procedures and equipment (some of which are bogus and dangerous) in recent years, programs that promote noninvasive, self-directed therapy often do nothing more than recycle the same old exercises and stretches seen in books and on websites, some decades old. Worse, they usually confuse exercise with stretching, without creating an action plan to deal with back pain and recovery. We decided it was time for an entirely new team approach.

Our goal with this book is to help anyone who's ever had lower back pain. We want to create a new mind-set for thinking about, using and strengthening your back—what we call Back Mindfulness.

One of the most important components of Back Mindfulness is for you to be aware at all times of how crucial your back is for every movement you make, and how you can't take it for granted any longer. After all, you want to get better and you know you need to get stronger, but you are afraid that in the process of getting stronger, you will hurt yourself. That's how Cara felt; anytime she did something physical, whether it was working out or cleaning her house, she was afraid of hurting herself but she was not mindful of her back until she was in pain. All of that has changed, and she has transformed her life into one that is free from lower back pain.

Another component of Back Mindfulness is that you need to see your lower back pain for what it really is—not just an annoyance, but an injury that must be treated, and treated properly. I'm convinced that one of the reasons why back pain is such a horrendous problem in this country is that the initial bouts of pain are often ignored or discounted because they're so common. Avoiding treatment, however, is what makes a small, easily managed injury become a major situation.

Once you start thinking about your back pain with the same level of seriousness that you'd think about a sprained wrist or a broken leg—injuries that you know you would treat promptly and properly—then you will do your utmost to respect the problem, manage the problem and prevent the problem from happening again. You will treat your back with the respect it deserves—and realize that proper treatment is not in the form of a pill. I particularly want to get you off any strong prescription medications you may have been given for your low back pain. Many of these meds have serious side effects and can become addictive. Why take them when you don't need them?

The 7-Minute Back Pain Solution is not just for those who have recurring back problems. It's for anyone who has the occasional twinge, wants a strong and supple core, wants to avoid back problems and/or wants to avoid surgery, and it's for those who have already had surgery. In other words, it's for everyone who wants to feel good, stand tall and strong, and not have to worry about back pain anymore.

HOW THE 7-MINUTE BACK PAIN SOLUTION WORKS

How many times have you said, "I can't do that. I just know I will hurt my back!" Wouldn't it be great *not* to have that fear anymore?

The 7-Minute Back Pain Solution will take that fear away, and it's incredibly easy to do, because you already have the equipment—your own muscles. We'll show you how to move them properly in a very short sequence of stretches that should be done at least once every day. Every time you stretch, this sequence should take no more than seven minutes to do. And these stretches have been uniquely designed so that they can be done safely by low back pain sufferers, even when the pain first hits.

When you start incorporating the 7-Minute Back Pain Solution into your daily life, you will:

Heal

By doing the seven stretches—which will take you only seven minutes—you will lengthen targeted muscles. When you do this, you release the tension they have created in your lower back.

Strengthen

Your core needs to be strong enough to support the weight of your entire body, and that's a big job! But we've found that many people don't understand what their "core" really is; usually, they assume it's only their abdominal muscles, most notably the rectus abdominis muscles in the upper abdomen, which get worked whenever you do crunches or sit-ups. These people have often erroneously been told that endless crunches will give them the six-pack of their dreams, but they don't realize that focusing on one part of the body to the detriment of another has a harmful effect. By overworking the abdominal muscles in the front, they ignore the corresponding muscles in their back, weakening them even as the demands put on them increase.

Actually, your core is not just about the muscles in the belly area of your abdomen—it encompasses all the muscles around your spine, hips and pelvis. When you incorporate specific exercises that target and strengthen your entire core, you create a powerful set of muscles that supports the areas of your back prone to aching.

The core-strengthening moves you'll find in Chapter 3 work the core in a far more effective way than traditional sit-ups. They strengthen the transverse abdominal (TVA) muscle, which is the deepest layer of the abdominal muscles, closest to your spine. The TVA acts as our body's internal girdle. When contracted, the TVA helps keep the spine and pelvis stable. This is incredibly effective at making sure you don't injure your back when you move.

Protect

Protection prevents intervention!

Improving the strength and power of your core will enable you to use all your other muscles properly, no matter what activity you have planned. This will make future bouts of severe pain and injuries much less likely. You'll be able to stop problems from happening.

Protection and prevention are not one-time things. They shouldn't be thought of as reactionary—in other words, as a reaction to a bout of acute pain. Instead, they need to be thought of as necessary to maintaining a healthy back. Cara and I stretch every day, and of course, we are not in pain every day. This daily stretching is like the "apple a day that keeps the doctor away"—it's the best protection we have for our backs.

Stretching is, of course, still a physical movement, even if it's one that you're putting your body through in order to help the healing process. Most of the clients Cara has stretched and trained through the years have commented on how careful she is when instructing and guiding them through these stretches and exercises. She knows it is her responsibility not only to teach her clients how to strengthen and stretch their bodies but to ensure that they protect themselves during any physical movement or activity. When you protect yourself, your chances of injury lessen, and you can then begin the healing process, because you will be able to take care of yourself without the risk. This book is all about showing you how to break that injury cycle!

Why Stretching?

Stretching will be discussed in much more detail in Chapters 1 and 2, but for now the most important concept to understand is what stretching actually is, and what it can do for your body. Stretching should not be thought of as "exercise" or a "workout." It's another activity altogether—one that should always complement your fitness routine. It's just as important for your body's overall health and fitness as what you commonly think of as exercise, or the kind of movement that makes you sweat and increases your heart rate.

HERE'S WHAT STRETCHING DOES:

- It maintains, improves and increases flexibility. Muscle flexibility allows your joints to move through their normal range of motion. A tight muscle can prevent your normal range of motion—which in turn can lead to an injury and pain.

- It lengthens the muscles and tendons, aiding in the prevention of injuries. By increasing the length and flexibility of your muscles through these stretches, less force is placed on the spine, and this, believe it or not, reduces the incidence of lower back pain.

- It aids in the repair of muscles and tendons, preventing soreness after exercise or sports.

- It increases the blood flow to the muscles, bringing them the nourishment they need while helping to remove waste and by-products. The better your blood flow to your muscles, the better your chances of a normal recovery from muscle and joint injury.

- It may slow the degeneration of muscles and joints.

- It often triggers the release of endorphins, those feel-good neuro-transmitters in your brain that are a wonderful stress reliever and your body's very own pain relief system.

- It helps you get a good night's sleep, as stretching before bed is not only relaxing but lengthens your muscles and helps with stiffness the next morning. This is especially important for those who find that spending many hours lying in bed makes their back pain worse. And, of course, a good night's rest is so important to your overall health and well-being.

- It improves your postural alignment. Tight muscles contribute to poor posture, while stretching makes muscles more flexible and less tight. With better posture when standing and sitting, you automatically reduce the pressure on your discs—causing you to hurt a lot less or not at all—and you stand taller and look leaner.

- It helps with balance and coordination, and thus has a positive impact on how you perform your regular daily activities.

When done properly, stretching should not compromise your back—which is a good thing! The stretches in this book have been specifically designed to lengthen your muscles while improving their flexibility, which is why you can do them even when you are in pain.

HERE'S WHAT STRETCHING CAN'T DO:

- It can't undo damage already done to the discs that cushion the bones of your spine.

IT IS EASY TO DO THESE STRETCHES:

- They take only a few minutes a day. We know that you have a finite amount of time every day, and life is busy. These stretches give you maximum results in minimal time. And if you choose to do them more than once each day, the benefits will quickly accrue.

- You don't need any equipment.

- With Cara as your guide, the photographs show you the proper form and technique for stretching, so you can learn how to protect yourself from future injuries.

- Anyone can stretch. Unless your physician specifically forbids it, you are rarely too old or too uncoordinated (an excuse Cara often hears) to do these kinds of stretches. You don't have to be a world-class athlete to become really good at stretching. You might not be able to master tennis or basketball, but you can always master stretching!

- Even if you are not in top physical condition, stretches work. For those in acute pain, they can even be done in bed or in a chair.

- Stretches can be done in your home or office, without you needing to change clothes. You do not need to go to a gym in order to have a great stretching routine. In fact, stretches can be done just about anywhere. We'll show you how to use your surroundings to improve your stretching. You'll see that if you brace yourself against something sturdy, you can usually stretch out a muscle or two and help your back pain go away.

HOW TO USE THIS BOOK

We created this system of stretches and core strengthening to be as practical and as user-friendly as possible. Before you start, of course, you must always see your physician or orthopedic specialist, especially if you have had bouts of back pain in the past or are in pain now, and have a thorough checkup. This assessment will rule out any of the potentially serious back issues, which may require surgical intervention. Once you know that your lower back pain is "common" (even if it is very painful) and you have been given the go-ahead by your physician to resume your regular activities, this is the book for you.

The information in this book is organized into two parts, because we have a two-pronged approach to managing and eradicating back pain.

Part I is all about the basics of the 7-Minute Back Pain Solution.

Chapter 1 teaches you the essentials about what causes back pain in the first place, and it also discusses back pain from a medical perspective, as well as treatment options for this pain.

Chapter 2 is the heart of the book—the how-to for the all-important stretches. We've broken down the stretches into easy-to-follow steps, and in the photographs you can see exactly how we want you to do them. Proper form and technique are crucial, so you won't have to worry about wasting your time and energy on useless movements.

Chapter 3 tackles the core strengthening exercises that will give your spine the support and protection it needs so you can stay out of pain.

The chapters in Part II give you extremely specific information about how to manage your daily life. The steps we show you will work whether you are still in pain, are in the healing process or have gotten rid of your pain. They'll make everything you do easier and less stressful on your back (and entire body). No matter the activity—from gardening to sitting at your desk to putting your baby in a car seat to buying shoes—you'll find strategies for doing it properly, no matter where you are. The instructions are concise and simple, and tell you precisely how to move when you are in pain, as well as how to protect yourself from future pain.

If your back pain persists, however, you might need more serious intervention. The Appendix gives you the information you need about noninvasive procedures, discusses whether or not you are a candidate for back surgery and outlines how to find an orthopedic surgeon in your area.

We compiled this information because many back-pain sufferers believe that they will always make their back pain worse by moving. However, they still need to take care of their homes and their families, and perform their job, so they must get up and go every day. It is difficult to really think about how to clean your house or sit in the car or carry groceries or set up your computer when your back is hurting. These are tasks we tend to do mindlessly.

We are going to show you *how to be mindful of your back at all times*. When you are, much to your astonishment, you soon realize that you are no longer trapped by back pain. You can minimize the risk. And instead of thinking about what you can't do, you'll see what you *can* do—which is basically just about everything!

Back Mindfulness is not, as you know by now, a one-time thing. It entails always thinking of your back first.

The 7-Minute Back Pain Solution is a system for life. Stretching is as essential as brushing your teeth, putting sunscreen on and drinking lots of water, and it takes just a little bit longer than these activities. It is also as essential as eating good food, getting some exercise, doing a good job at work, laughing and loving. Consider it one of your daily functions for optimum health. Once you do, as soon as you feel any back pain, you won't panic or reach for the pain pills that knock you flat out. You won't need to rush to the doctor or wonder how you'll manage a two-hour drive. You'll know exactly what to do to make the pain go away.

In a way, Back Mindfulness is like dance training, only on a much different scale. It might help to think about why professional ballet dancers go to class every day, even though they could do the steps in their sleep. It's the sheer repetitiveness of the exercises over time that makes them second nature—and enables dancers to perform intricate choreography without having to worry about the *how*. They're able to do it because their muscles instantly respond to commands from their brain.

When done over time, these stretches, as well as the core exercises, will become second nature to you, too. This is why you'll see the instructions to "contract your abdominals" so often. Mindful contractions create memories and connections in your brain, so you'll soon be doing them automatically. Not only will your muscles become longer, stronger and more flexible, but you won't have to think it through when you need to make any kind of movement. You will move your body to maximize its own power—and at the same time you'll keep your back stable and protected.

Let us empower you while we show you how easy it is to transform your daily routine so you can avoid the back pain that has made your life a misery.

The 7-Minute Back Pain Solution is proof that small can actually be big: the small and simple changes you make to your daily routine will have benefits so large that the back pain that has made your life a misery will be no more than a fading memory of what used to be and will be no longer.

You *can* conquer back pain. It is *not* going to conquer you!

Bad Back Myths

Please don't believe that any of these are true!

1. The severity of back pain means the severity of the outcome. In other words, truly debilitating back pain—the kind that makes it

an agony to move—means my injury is serious and dangerous and will lead to chronic problems and/or surgery.

2. If I move when low back pain hits, I will do severe damage.

3. When my back hurts, lying on a bed or couch will help it.

4. Having low back pain means I will be disabled.

5. If I don't get some form of ongoing professional treatment for my back pain, it will become chronic.

6. My back pain is not from an injury.

7. The pain will go away by itself.

8. If my lower back hurts, it always means I've damaged my nerves.

9. If I have damaged my nerves, this damage will be permanent.

10. Back pain is caused by me spraining my muscles.

11. Low back pain is caused by arthritis.

12. Once my back goes out, I'm doomed. I'll have to worry about this kind of pain for the rest of my life.

13. Low back pain is hereditary. If either or both of my parents had it, I'm going to have it, too.

14. If my back is hurting, I can't have sex.

15. If my back is hurting, I can't exercise at all.

16. If I do start feeling better with professional treatment, I'll heal right away.

17. Only overweight people have problems with their back.

18. Only out-of-shape people have problems with their back.

19. Doing sit-ups or crunches is the only way to make my back stronger.

20. An X-ray of my back will clearly show where the problem is.

21. I have to think about dealing with my back only when it hurts.

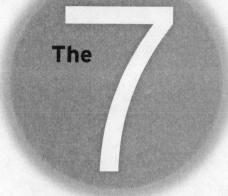

The 7

MINUTE
BACK PAIN
SOLUTION

PART

I

Why Your Back Hurts, and How to Stretch and Strengthen Your Back

CHAPTER 1

BACK PAIN BASICS

LOUISE WAS SITTING IN MY OFFICE, looking anxious. A forty-four-year-old working mother of two, she spent her weekdays at an office and her weekends driving the kids around to a variety of activities. Her back had started aching one bright Sunday, over ten days earlier, after she helped a group of kids clamber up into her minivan after soccer practice.

"When I lifted the soccer bag, I felt a big sort of bad twinge in my back," she told me. "So when I got home, I went right to the medicine cabinet and took some of my leftover pain meds from my recent dental surgery. I stayed in bed the rest of the day, but the pills didn't really help. The next day the pain was so bad, I couldn't go to work. I was lucky my mom was able to come and take care of the kids after school, but I missed a whole week of work, and now my boss is mad at me, because he thinks I'm faking, and my kids are mad at me because I was hurt too bad to pay any attention to them, and my husband is mad because I couldn't do what I usually do around the house." She burst into tears. "And the pain just won't go away. I can't take it anymore."

Louise was a typical patient with low back pain. And like most of my typical patients, she unwittingly made things worse after she felt that initial twinge:

- She didn't know how to treat the pain, so she took prescription meds that were not prescribed for this problem (something no one should *ever* do!).

- She stayed in bed.

- She hoped the pain would go away by itself.

After I examined Louise and ruled out anything serious, I told her that her pain was due to back strain—and that what had happened to her was not her fault. In fact, it was incredibly common. And I told her that I was giving her permission to *move* so she could get back to her normal activities.

Like most patients who hear this information, she looked at me in shock. "But I'm afraid to move. It hurts too much!" she said. "Won't that make things worse?"

"No, it won't," I told her. "It will help you heal." Then I sent her home with instructions on how to do the 7-Minute Back Pain Solution stretches and told her that if she didn't get better after doing them for several weeks, only then might she be a candidate for a more intense workup.

Louise was very relieved, especially when I told her that she didn't need to see me again if her back got better—but to expect that to take several weeks, at the very least.

WHY IS BACK PAIN SO COMMON?

Louise was glad to know that her back pain wasn't unique, and I explained to her that there are many reasons why our backs hurt so much. Here are the most common:

- You sit all day long. And guess what? The worst possible position for your back is a seated position. Yet most workers spend 90 percent of their time in a chair in a non-ergonomic workplace. And they drive a car to and from work. Add to the mix that 90 percent of adults over twenty-one years of age have a job. You do the math! We're talking hundreds of millions of people.

- You don't think or care about taking optimal care of your back until it hurts, and yet when it hurts, you're too afraid to move (which inadvertently makes things worse).

- You aren't in good physical shape.

- You're trying to get in shape, but you can sometimes be a weekend warrior and you can't help but overdo it. This sets up a cycle where you work out too hard, have pain, stop working out, then go right back to the gym or your favorite sport and start hurting again ... and so on!

- You do work out regularly, but you often push yourself too hard, sometimes working out or playing sports even when you're in pain.

- You rarely, if ever, do the kind of exercises that strengthen all your core muscles properly.

- You rarely, if ever, stretch your muscles after a workout, and even if you know you should, you don't, because you don't have the time.

- You love your high heels or shoes that look fabulous but don't quite fit properly.

- You're always on the go, carrying heavy bags or children or both, and then cleaning the house and doing the daily chores for your family.

- You know you aren't in shape, but as soon as there's snow in the driveway, you're out there shoveling.

- It happens!

The good news, of course, is that once you add a regular stretching routine to your daily life, and once you strengthen the core muscles that support your spine, you will not only alleviate your low back pain but also help prevent recurring bouts of it. Like all good machines, you need to warm up your spine and condition your muscles before becoming a champion at what you do, whether it's swimming at the Y, taking care of the garden, running after your kids or playing eighteen holes of golf as a weekend warrior.

So why are backs so prone to bouts of debilitating pain, and how can stretching really help? In order to understand why stretching is so beneficial for back-pain sufferers, you first need to understand a bit about the unique anatomy of your spine and the muscles that surround it. What, precisely, does your "back" entail? What are the normal structures found within, and what can go wrong, and where? Why is the pain so terrible, and what triggers it in the first place?

In the next section, I'll first discuss the basics of your spine's anatomy, showing you how it works in terms of its different components, such as the discs, and in conjunction with the muscles that surround it and comprise your core. Once you see how all these components fit together and work synergistically, it's much easier to visualize what can go wrong, and then figure out how to manage it with the seven-minute stretches you'll learn about in Chapter 2.

UNDERSTANDING YOUR BACK

The unique anatomy of our spines enables us to bend, sit, twist, dance, run, hop, swim, make love and lean over the crib railing to kiss our babies good night. But we pay for this amazing flexibility, as it also makes it incredibly easy for low back pain to strike.

The Three Sections of Your Spine

Your spinal column is strong and flexible, yet fragile at the same time. How's that for paradoxical?

The spine is made up of bones, muscles, ligaments, joints, nerves, discs and the spinal cord. There are twenty-four vertebrae in your spine, which are in place to house and protect the nerves of your spinal cord found within, and they're cushioned by spongy discs that provide support and spacing for the nerves. Your lower body and your spine are supported by large muscle groups called the paraspinal muscles or erecti muscles of the back. These muscles encase the vertebrae and aid in the range of motion of your spine.

THERE ARE THREE SECTIONS OF YOUR SPINE:

- The cervical spine is located in the area of your neck that connects your skull to your shoulder area. There are seven cervical vertebrae, aligned in a reverse C shape to give your neck the proper contour. The vertebrae are numbered C1–C7.

The Three Sections of Your Spine

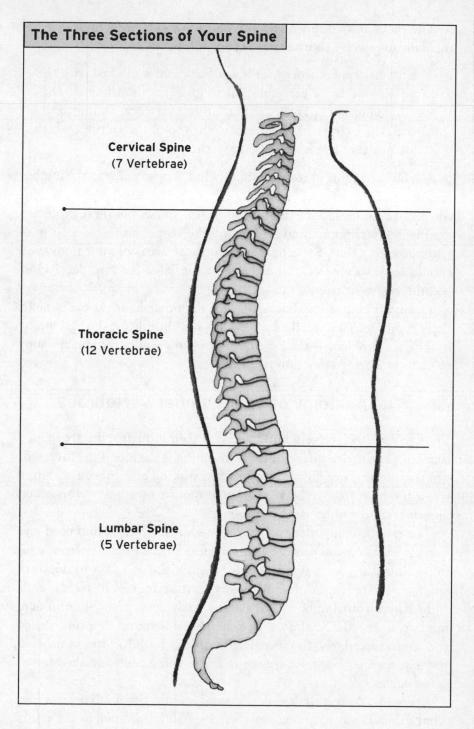

Cervical Spine
(7 Vertebrae)

Thoracic Spine
(12 Vertebrae)

Lumbar Spine
(5 Vertebrae)

- The thoracic spine anchors your rib cage and is fairly immobile. There are twelve thoracic vertebrae, numbered T1–T12.

- The lumbar spine forms your lower back and is aligned with the same contour as the cervical spine to give that nice shape to the small of your back. There are five lumbar vertebrae, numbered L1–L5. The L5 vertebra connects to the top of the sacrum, which is composed of five bones fused together.

As you know, this book is all about what happens only to the lumbar region and its five vertebrae. There can be pain in and problems with the cervical spine and the thoracic spine, of course, but these problems are much less common and are beyond the scope of this book. It goes without saying that if you have pain in those areas of your body, you should see your physician or orthopedic specialist for a proper diagnosis and treatment plan.

Lumbar pain, or low back pain, on the other hand, is overwhelmingly common. This small area is what's responsible for the vast majority of back problems—the kind that can leave you in too much agony to go to work or to function properly.

The Anatomy of Your Lumbar Vertebrae

The five vertebrae, or vertebral bodies, of your lumbar spine are shaped like cunning little square boxes. The spine is divided into three columns: anterior, middle and posterior. Looking at a person standing sideways, from front to back, these columns are arranged in this order: anterior, middle, posterior.

The middle component of your spine houses your spinal cord and nerves. This is nerve central, transmitting all the impulses from your brain down to your muscles and limbs. But the spinal cord does not span the entire length of your twenty-four vertebrae. In fact, it ends right where your lumbar spine begins, at what's called the thoracic-lumbar junction. The end of the spinal cord is found in a tube called the conus medularis. In most people, this is found in the same area, namely, the mid-back, where the thoracic spine ends and the lumbar spine begins.

The spinal cord itself does not descend into the five lumbar vertebrae; what's found instead are numerous nerve rootlets known as the cauda

The Anatomy of Your Lumbar Vertebrae

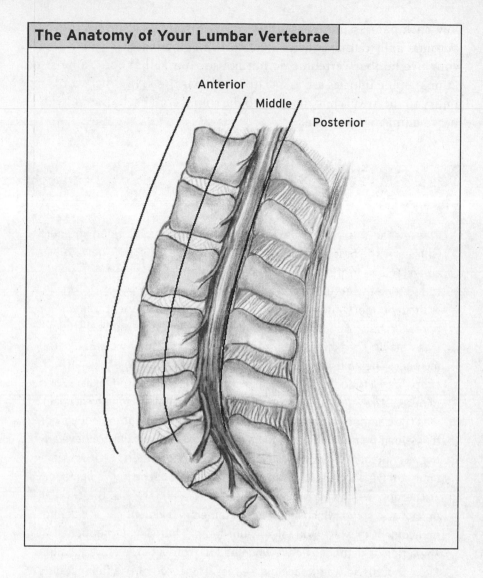

Anterior

Middle

Posterior

equina, often called "the horse's tail," because that's what it resembles. The cauda equina functions to stimulate your lower extremities. Think of it as a sort of electrical box, sending out signals to different parts of your body. Because we know which nerves in the spine affect which muscles in your body, when you have pain in certain muscles, we can pinpoint which area of your spine is responsible for it.

It is extremely important to understand the difference between the spinal cord and the spinal nerve rootlets, because most people with low back pain assume that if they move or twist in any way, they will automatically damage their spinal cord. Let me reassure you. Because your five lumbar vertebrae do not house your spinal cord, almost no lumbar spine injuries are associated with paralysis. In other words, an injury to the area is not an injury to the spinal cord itself. But individual nerve damage is possible.

Low Back Pain and Its Treatment Will *Never* Leave You Paralyzed!

Please read this sidebar before you move on, because when you hurt your back, the first thought you usually have is, *Oh no, I will never move again*. This fear of paralysis is so common and sometimes more debilitating than the actual back pain itself.

I truly understand my patients' fears about permanent damage or paralysis, because I've been there myself. When I was a medical student, I was playing basketball with some classmates one night and twisted my back. The pain was incredibly intense, and I felt an electric jolt with every step. I thought for sure I had herniated, or ruptured, a disc. For a minute I stood absolutely still, worried about what I'd done to my back. Was the damage severe? Instead, what I was feeling was my body's normal (albeit painful) response to an unfortunate twist. I did not have any nerve damage. I did not cause any nerve damage when I kept walking—I might have aggravated my injury, but I did *not* cause nerve damage.

The only way to become paralyzed is from an injury to the cervical or thoracic spine, which might be sustained in a violent car accident or an accident in which you fall on your head. That is what happened to the actor Christopher Reeve when he fell from a horse during a jump. Even though he was wearing a helmet, the force of the fall instantly compressed his neck vertebrae and cracked them, leaving him a quadriplegic.

Even after I carefully explain this to many of my patients, they still are often very fearful that surgery to the lumbar region is going to paralyze them, even though that is physiologically impossible. The absolute worst-case scenario would be a loss of function of an individual nerve, which is still highly unlikely.

The Motion Segments of Your Vertebrae

Most people think that low back pain is caused by a strain or stress to the muscles surrounding the spine. Instead, it is really a strain or stress to the spinal motion segment, which in turn triggers the nearby muscles to go into protective mode. This means they get inflamed— and you'll see what I mean by spinal "inflammation" in the section on p. 26—which in turn increases their stress load. This is what causes the debilitating pain.

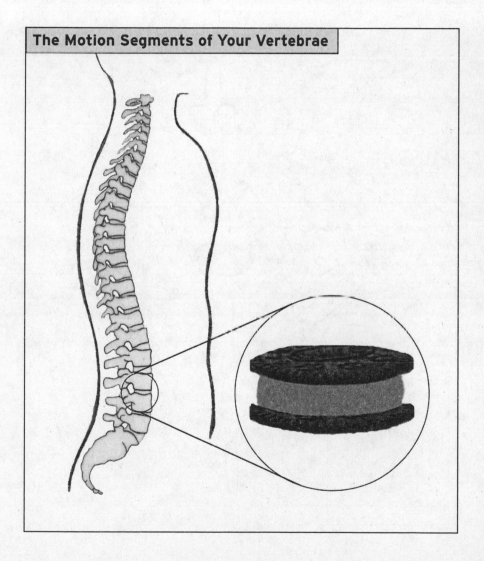

The Motion Segments of Your Vertebrae

There are five motion segments in the lumbar spine. Each consists of a vertebral body, a soft disc in the middle and another vertebral body, and two joints (or facets). One motion segment is comprised of two facets and one disc, forming a tripod. Think of a motion segment as your spine's equivalent of an Oreo cookie, with the disc being the cream and the vertebral bodies the chocolate cookie.

Facets of the Spine

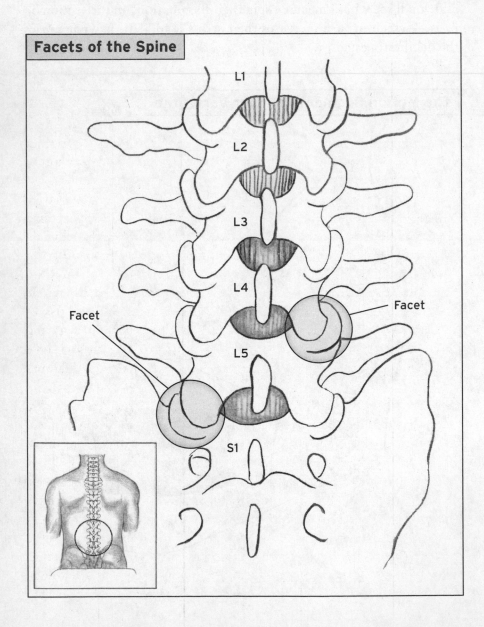

The joint's facets are freely moveable synovial joints, similar to what's found in your knee. In other words, the facet is the joint, and the motion segment is a combination of the vertebral body, disc and facets. Yet while the joints of each lumbar vertebra form a joint, they don't protect each other. If one segment gets injured, this affects the other segments.

Your facets can become injured when you inadvertently hyperextend your back (or push it past its normal range of motion), lift or pick up something wrong, shovel wrong, clean your kitchen wrong, or for no reason at all.

All About Discs

Spinal discs are made up of collagen and water, and they are sandwiched between the bones of your spine to add support and aid in motion. A single disc looks like a sunny-side-up egg, with a nucleus pulposus in the center as its yolk, surrounded by lamellae, made of layers and layers of water and thicker collagen fibers, which hold everything in place. Healthy discs provide height to the motion segments, allowing for more room for the nerves, and they serve as a shock absorber for your entire spine.

Spinal discs are really marvelous creations. They are avascular, meaning that they do not have a blood supply, as other cells and tissues do. Instead, discs rely on an osmotic gradient that works by gravity and flow. When you lie down, the discs swell and allow nutrients to come in; when you stand up, the discs do a sort of little swish, which allows the waste to come out.

In other words, discs rely on gravity and movement to remove waste materials. This is what keeps them healthy. Obviously, staying prone in bed for long periods makes this process impossible—which is one of the reasons why bed rest is antithetical to healing low back pain!

A healthy, normal disc is fully enclosed, but if it gets damaged, micro-tearing will allow some of the water content to leak out. Think of how the yolk of a sunny-side egg loses its shape when your fork slices through it. A damaged disc leaks fluid, and this fluid in turn affects the nerves, causing more nerve endings to form—and more nerves means more pain. In addition, the disc loses height and shrinks. As it does, nerve endings form in these micro-tears. As you know, nerves are what

Normal Lumbar Intervertebral Disc

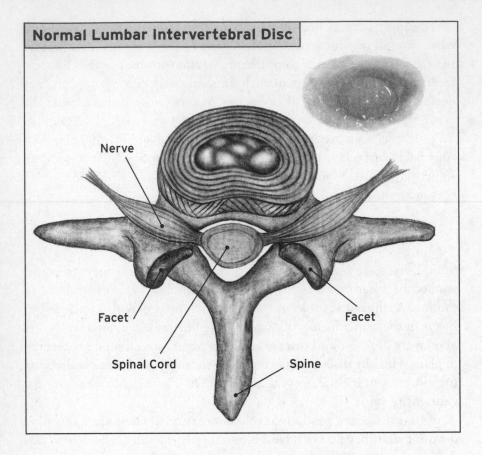

Nerve

Facet

Facet

Spinal Cord

Spine

allow you to feel pain. This entire process is like vines in a garden growing when you don't want them to and where you don't want them to—as these new nerves in your lower back grow into the micro-tears and form a pain generator.

This process is called disc degeneration. It is not like joint deterioration or even brain deterioration. It is not arthritis, which is inflammation of the joints and surrounding tissues. While an injury can lead to disc degeneration, for some people, degenerative discs are genetically determined, meaning they were born with this predisposition.

Disc degeneration is not necessarily age related. It's very important to understand that you can have a degenerative disc when you're twenty or when you're eighty. Disc damage often happens to young athletes who push themselves, who don't understand the importance of stretching and good core training, or who may have overzealous coaches, resulting in extremely painful and sometimes life-changing over-use injuries. This is very frustrating for me as there's no reason for teenagers or young adults to be pushed to the point of serious disc damage.

Or you might be a weekend warrior who thinks that it's no problem to suit up and go outside and run a few miles, and you don't factor in

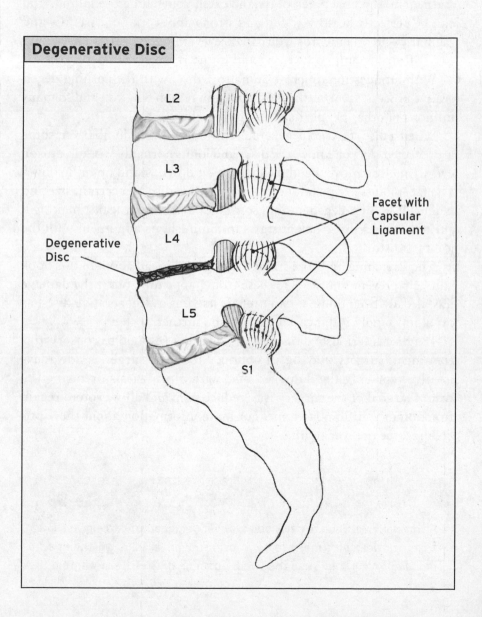

Degenerative Disc

L2

L3

Facet with
Capsular
Ligament

Degenerative
Disc

L4

L5

S1

any stretching or warming up, or you don't consider how crucial it is to gradually build up your strength and endurance. Good intentions are great; not knowing how to ease into exercise is not!

That said, injuries or micro-trauma to your discs can happen with almost absurd ease. You might pick something up the wrong way, twist too far when hitting a golf ball, sit too long when you're stuck in a traffic jam, slip on a patch of ice and catch yourself before falling. You can be perfectly healthy and fit and strong and work out carefully and regularly—in other words, you can do everything right—and back pain can still strike with no warning and for no reason whatsoever!

Without question, micro-trauma to a disc, with the ensuing degenerative process, is by far the most common reason why you and so many millions of other people have low back pain.

When a disc starts to degenerate, the joints in your lumbar vertebrae are affected. As you know, the discs and joints normally work in unison every time you move, bend, flex, twist, sit down, stand up or lie down. The facet joints are positioned to work with a disc of a certain size and height. With disc degeneration, some of a disc's water leaks, making it shrink. Once a disc's height starts to diminish, its alignment with the joints is disturbed.

The stretching and core strengthening you'll read about in this book can help prevent injuries like these from happening, but if the damage has already been done, it can't repair itself as a degenerative disc has no blood supply. All it can do is degrade further.

If a disc is seriously damaged and does not respond to conservative treatment, surgery may be an option. Most disc surgeries nowadays involve replacing the damaged disc with a prosthesis or fusing the disc. The goal of the surgery is to reduce pain and allow you to regain function in your lumbar spine. For more information about these procedures, see the Appendix.

Will Losing Weight Help Your Back?

All my patients who are a few pounds overweight automatically assume that their weight is a major factor causing their back pain. Will their back pain improve if they shed the twenty pounds they've been wanting to lose? No! I have plenty of patients with lower back pain whose body mass index (or BMI) is extremely high, but I also have many patients with lower back pain who are skinny, with a weight way below a normal BMI. Back pain can strike anyone. Having a high BMI doesn't automatically mean you'll have back problems.

But if you lose those twenty pounds and get in better shape—especially if you add stretching and core strengthening to your daily routine—you should hopefully see and feel a noticeable difference in your cardiovascular health and your blood sugar levels, and experience other health benefits.

The Muscles of Your Back—It's All About the Core

Your core has many different muscles, which help you move and which protect and keep your spine stable when you do so. Whether you are prone to back pain or not, you'll want to have a back whose muscles are as strong as possible. Without strong muscles, you automatically increase your risk for suffering from back pain in the future, because if your core is weak, this will result in a body that responds poorly to the regular daily demands placed upon it.

We can't emphasize enough how important it is to do everything in your power to strengthen all your core muscles. After all, how well your back functions is crucial to practically every movement you make. You don't get up out of bed at the impetus of your feet or knees or arms or head—you get up because your brain sends the necessary signals through your spinal column, and your back muscles kick into gear and allow you to move.

After seventeen years as a spine surgeon, and after seeing thousands and thousands of patients, I can tell you that at their initial office visit almost none of my patients have any idea what it actually means to strengthen their core muscles. They think that their "core" is centered in the front of their body, in the abdomen, and that the back muscles have little to do with it. Because of this erroneous belief, they assume that the best way to make their core stronger is to get down on the floor and start (and then end) with crunches or sit-ups every day. They are almost always astonished when I tell them that crunches work predominately on the rectus abdominis muscles, which are but a small part of all the muscles that comprise your entire core. This makes the crunch an inefficient exercise for the overall strengthening of your core.

The Muscles of Your Core

Rectus Abdominis, External Obliques, Internal Obliques, Transverse Abdominis, Erector Spinae, Multifidus, Hip Flexors (Psoas Major, Iliacus, Rectus Femoris, Pectineus and Sartorius), Gluteus Medius, Gluteus Minimus, Gluteus Maximus, Hamstrings, Piriformis, Hip Adductors, Pelvic Floor Muscles.

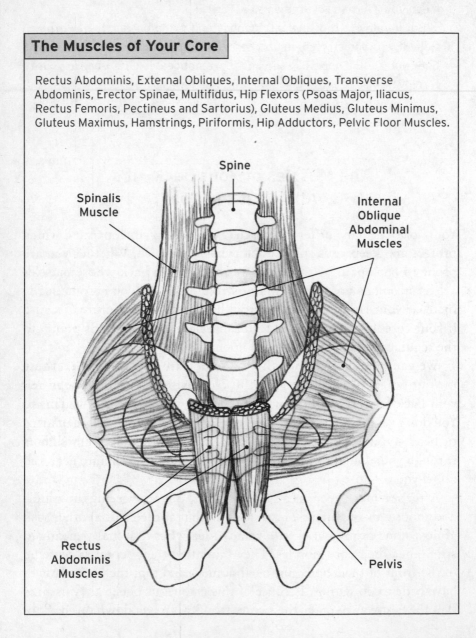

Spine

Spinalis Muscle

Internal Oblique Abdominal Muscles

Rectus Abdominis Muscles

Pelvis

You Need a Strong Core

Because so many people think their core is composed only of their abdominal muscles, they do those endless crunches, with perhaps a few twists to the side to work their obliques, and then wonder why their back still hurts.

The reason is simple: your core is not just about flat abdominal muscles—it's about *all* the many muscles that encircle your entire torso. These include the abdominal, side, hip and back muscles. Instead of thinking of your core as a flat surface, like you hope your belly will be after you do hundreds of sit-ups, you should instead think of it as a three-dimensional circle or sphere.

In addition to your rectus abdominis muscles, which are strengthened by sit-ups and crunches, the core includes your oblique muscles, which run along each side of your body; the transverse abdominal muscle and the multifidus muscle, which are close to your spine and are especially important in unison as they help to stabilize your spine when you move to protect yourself from injury; the extensor muscles, which are located in the small of your back; and the hip flexors, which attach to your pelvis. All these muscles attach to the lumbar spine, and their primary functions are to allow bending, flexing and rotation, and to aid the spine in all its motions.

These muscles don't just work on their own, though, in isolation, and therefore when you work muscles on one side of your core, you also need to work those on the other side. That's because muscles like these are meant to function synergistically. There's always going to be an agonist/antagonist response; that's how muscles work. When one muscle does more of the work than its corresponding muscle, the neglected muscle becomes weakened. Overcompensation by one set of muscles at the expense of the opposing set is what causes muscle imbalance.

For example, your biceps are located in the front of your arm, above your elbow, and they are responsible for flexing your arm. Your triceps are located in the back of your arm, attached to your elbow, and are responsible for extending your arm. Just as you work both muscles in your arm to keep balance, you need to work your abdominal muscles along with the erector muscles. This will balance your core.

Or consider what happens to us when we sit. Our hip flexors, hamstrings (found at the back of your thighs) and quadriceps (found at the front of your thighs) become tight, and our abdominal and gluteus muscles in our buttocks become soft and weak. When the hip flexors, hamstrings and quadriceps become tight, they shorten in length; this pulls your pelvis out of alignment, either forward or backward.

The same situation is found with your core muscles. If you work on the abdominal muscles in your front while neglecting the muscles in the back, you will create an imbalance. Your back muscles can't possibly be as strong and will need to work that much harder to compensate for their weakness. When these back muscles are strained to their limit, you will, unfortunately, know about it instantly!

Getting to the Core of Sit-ups and Crunches

Who doesn't want a flat, toned, sculpted stomach, commonly called a six-pack? The truth about attaining those chiseled muscles, however, is that it's often out of your control. Genetics plays a large part in your anatomy, so if your parents did not have a sculpted abdominal region even if they exercised well, you might not be able to have one, either. Six-packs are also a function of what and how much you eat, how many calories you expend and your body fat distribution.

When performing a crunch or a sit-up, you are working the rectus abdominis and oblique muscles (agonists) without engaging any corresponding back muscles (antagonists). As a result, the agonist/antagonist muscles are unbalanced. You need to strengthen your back muscles as much as your six-pack muscles! In addition, when proper form is not used, the hip flexor muscles can take over, meaning they become dominant and do most of the work. That is often why so many people say they can do countless crunches yet not really feel it where they should—in their abdominals. You can better maximize your exercise time by doing the core exercises in Chapter 3.

This abdominal muscles/back muscles imbalance can create a vicious cycle: having weak abdominal muscles makes it more difficult for you to strengthen your back muscles, but if your back muscles are weak, they will often feel very tight. This tightness then causes pain in your lower back, making you disinclined to do any stretches or exercises that you think are going to cause more pain. Breaking this cycle and getting you out of pain are what this book is all about. First we'll get you out of pain with the seven stretches, and then you'll strengthen your core muscles in a safe way that will not compromise your back. This will prevent the cycle from starting all over again.

A strong core will also aid in improving your posture, which is incredibly important. You'll be able to stand more erect and walk for longer periods of time, or even lean over a computer or sit in your office without discomfort. That's because a powerful core also helps with what's called a neutral spine position. This is the basic curve of your spine from your head down through your waist, and includes the cervical, thoracic and lumbar spine. It's the normal and natural curve of your spine and is an **S** shape. An ideal neutral spine position is one where all three curves in the **S** shape are present. The position should not cause pain and it should actually minimize your lower back pain, acting as a sort of cushion to protect your spine from the normal or extraordinary demands you might put on it.

You always want to strive to have a neutral spine position, no matter what task you're doing, or whether you're hard at work or relaxing after a stressful day. And the way to do that is with strong, flexible, well-balanced muscles. Weak abdominal muscles tighten up the hip flexor muscles, pulling the pelvis forward; too-tight hamstrings will pull the pelvis back. The result, as you know, can be lower back pain.

Since everyone has a slightly different **S** shape to their bodies, it's impossible to standardize a basic neutral spine position. You'll know what yours is when your strong core improves your posture and muscle strength. When you maintain the neutral spine position throughout your day, you allow your body to perform most efficiently and effectively. Stretching your tightened-up muscles and strengthening your core muscles are the easiest things you can do to achieve and maintain an ideal neutral spine position.

A strong core and an ideal neutral spine position ensure that both men and women have a more satisfying sex life, as they are able to function better sexually. You won't just look good; you'll feel good, too.

A Good Core Workout Should Be an Essential Part of Every Workout

Strengthening your entire core should always be part of every workout. You'll reap the benefits in every possible way. When you have a strong core, *everything* you do will be better, and not just in the gym or when you play a sport. All muscle movements originate with the core. If the core is strong, you will perform all activities better.

For example, if a weight lifter wants big, bulky biceps yet has a weak core, every time he wants to pull up that weight, it will be difficult for him without the powerful muscles that form the foundation for muscle movement and strength. If, on the other hand, his core is powerful, he will not find himself struggling to lift.

If you incorporate the stretches in this book, along with the strengthening core exercises that you'll find in Chapter 3, and strengthen your core, even if you develop pain, it should be on a lesser scale, with a shorter recuperation time. You should also have fewer recurrences.

THE MEDICAL TREATMENT OF BACK PAIN

Years ago I had a patient named Claire, who really made me think about the nature of chronic pain. She told me that she knew it was extremely far-fetched, but that one of her biggest anxieties was that a fire would start in her home when she was alone and her back was out. What would she do if she literally couldn't move faster than a very slow crawl or get up from bed? Could she get to the phone? Could she hurry down the stairs and out the door? Her worry was that she would not be able to move and function at her normal speed in an emergency situation.

Claire was a perfect example of how fear can paralyze you even when back pain will not. I tried to reassure her that quick movements—like rushing to get out of the house if a fire has started—would not cause permanent damage, but it took a lot of coaxing to help her move past her terror. When you're in pain, your mind often doesn't let you see the pain for what it is: something that can eventually leave your body just as easily as it arrived.

What finally freed Claire from these worries was learning how to do the stretches in this book. She realized that *she* could take control over her back pain, instead of having it control her.

More Than Anything, Realize That the Pain Is Usually Worse than What Caused It

Back pain is often absolutely agonizing, debilitating and torturous. But that doesn't mean your injury is as severe as the pain you feel. In other words, the amount of pain is *not* directly proportional to the injury itself. You can truly suffer from the worst back pain of your life, yet what caused it can be incredibly minor and easy to fix.

I know this might be hard to believe at first—because back pain is often so overwhelmingly torturous—but it really is true. Severe low back pain does *not* necessarily mean severe injury. It doesn't necessarily mean you need expensive long-term treatment, like physical therapy or surgery. It doesn't mean you need a prescription for heavy-duty, potentially addictive narcotics.

And it certainly doesn't mean that you are doomed to a lifetime of more pain. But when the pain is so all-encompassing, it can be very difficult *not* to believe that it automatically means you have a really horrible, huge problem to deal with.

The Real Reasons Why You Have Back Pain

Carl was sitting in my office, looking and feeling miserable. "It's the sitting that kills me, Doc," he said. "I was at the movies the other day with my wife, and my back started hurting. I was fidgeting and squirming and rubbing it because I couldn't get comfortable. Then, when I stood up, the pain was so bad, I nearly passed out."

Carl had suffered a classic episode of low back pain, one that had been brewing for quite some time. He didn't work out as often as he should, and he had weak core muscles. He never stretched. He drove a lot for his job, and when he was back in his office, he had to sit in the chair that was given to him, like all the other employees. So that extra sitting in a crummy movie theater chair was the last straw, putting extra pressure on an area that was about to snap. He injured his disc, and his muscles seized up in response. But Carl couldn't do much about it when the pain struck. He still had to get up, walk down the stairs, get into his car (luckily, his wife could get the car and pull it up to the front of the theater) and get back home, where he spent all night in pain, worrying about how he would manage his workweek.

An analogy I like to use is this: parents of a young baby or child who suddenly spikes a fever are often in a panic. They do whatever it takes to bring the fever down, often not realizing that the fever is not the underlying illness, but a symptom of it. Well, back pain is like having a fever. The pain is not the main problem—the pain is a *response* to it. For whatever reason, your back has seized up, and your body is clever enough to send out pain signals, telling you to slow down so you can take care of yourself and heal.

But do most people know how to slow down and heal? No, they do not. That's because they do not think of their back pain as an injury. If these people had sprained an ankle, they would do the right thing. They'd go to their doctor or the emergency room for X-rays to make sure their ankle wasn't broken. They'd put ice on the site to reduce swelling. They'd listen to their doctor's diagnosis and follow the advice given, and they'd stay off that leg for as long as they were told to. They would know they had an injury and that it must be managed properly in order to heal well.

Well, when you are suddenly hit with back pain, that is also an injury. But because you can't see it—and because you might still be able to move, albeit painfully, whereas with a sprained ankle you literally can't put any weight on your foot—you may not take this bout of pain as seriously as you should. This is an enormous problem, because every time you have an episode, or flare, of back pain, it is due to an *injury*. Yet if you dismiss the injury to your lower back, how can you treat it properly? How can you help it heal with maximum speed and minimal pain?

Most of my patients have told me that the first thing they do when they have back pain is lie down on the sofa or their bed. Yet this is the very worst thing you can do—because it sets up a vicious cycle. Lying down makes your tight muscles tighten up even more, making the situation worse. And the more you do that without getting to the root of what's making you tight, the harder it is to break the cycle.

When you have typical lower back pain, yes, you have an injury. But you have not injured or sprained the muscles surrounding your spine in the same way that you can sprain a joint, like your ankle or knee. Instead, as you know from the first few sections of this chapter, you have injured some element in your spine—the facet joints or the discs—and there is a cascading response. Orthopedists call this discogenic back pain, mechanical back pain or facet pain. This is what happens:

- Your body goes on high alert. Something has happened, and the spine needs to be protected.

- The facet joints have nerves around them to react to stimuli. The muscles attached to the spine and facet joints work in unison to allow normal motion. When there is an adverse signal or trauma to the area, these muscles can freeze up, and this will stop normal motion.

- When these stimulating signals from your nerves arrive, the muscle's response is to tighten up.

- As you know, muscles are made up of many different interconnected fibers. When they tighten up, the contraction causes intense pain.

- The pain can spread as more muscles get the signals to contract and tighten, leading to a buildup of inflammation in the muscles, which gives off a noxious stimulus, or an irritant. The pain can then spread to your joints.

Bottom line: when back pain comes on, it is due to your muscles tightening up *in response* to an injury.

As bad as it may be, think of the pain as a kind of short circuit or safety catch. This intense, debilitating sensation is your body's safety catch, telling all the little nerve endings in your muscles that they're on notice that extreme care must be taken in order for the injury to heal. If you had no pain, you'd never know that you'd been injured, and you could end up with far worse damage.

Notice that I said "extreme care"—I didn't say you shouldn't move at all! This is why it is so important to stretch your muscles. Stretching is what gets the tightened-up muscles to disengage and release the tightness. Stretching will literally reset your system, stopping the cascade effect on your muscles in its tracks.

Back Pain and Inflammation

I believe one of the reasons some people are terrified that back pain instantly means disability or paralysis is that when they hear the word "inflammation," they think "swollen." And if they're swollen up, with fluid pressing on the spine and nerves, then they're in serious trouble, right?

"Inflammation" is a term that many people use when talking about low back pain, but it's one that few understand. But that's okay, because it is confusing!

Inflammation is a complex biological response of vascular tissues in your body to a harmful stimulus. This can come in the form of trauma to a joint or trauma to muscles, tendons and ligaments. The inflammation that comes after the trauma is your body's protective attempt to remove the harmful stimulus and to initiate the healing process.

Inflammation can be classified as acute or chronic. Acute inflammation is your body's initial response to whatever has harmed it, and there is a cascade of biochemical events involving blood cells, immune cells and various other cells within the injured tissue. Blood flow to the damaged area also increases. This means that the injured area can become very swollen due to what is called vasodilation, when the blood vessels open and numerous cells flow into the area, wall it off and are then involved in repairing the injury. This is a biochemical response, and swelling is seen with trauma-type injuries to joints, such as the knee and ankle.

This kind of inflammation, however, is *not* the same as what happens with lower back pain. Lower back pain or muscle strain happens when your muscle fibers are abnormally stretched or torn. Lumbar strain also happens when the ligaments, the tough bands of tissues that hold the bones together, are torn from their attachment. (Differentiating a strain from a sprain can be difficult as these injuries show similar symptoms.)

To reiterate, inflammation in a muscle is not the same as inflammation in a joint. If you have lower back pain or strain from an injury, there is a slight disruption of the muscle fibers, which triggers an inflammatory response in the muscle, which induces even more muscle soreness. Much of this soreness is due to a buildup of by-products that are formed from the initial injury, predominately lactic acid, which is highly caustic. These by-products prevent the muscles from working properly and act as noxious stimuli, irritating them and impeding the normal flow of nicely oxygenated red blood cells to the area, which are needed to clear out the substances that have built up.

Stretching is extremely important in this initial phase of muscle inflammation as it aids in the prevention of chronic damage to the erecti muscles of your back. Stretching, massage therapy, physical therapy and exercise all increase the normal blood flow to the muscles, speeding along the clearing out or cleansing of these noxious by-products. This allows your muscles to rejuvenate and regain their normal state. Increased blood flow also brings cells to the muscles to help repair these muscle strains or sprains.

Why Massage Helps Low Back Pain

Many of my new patients who slowly walk into my office hold their back with their hand, applying pressure and hoping the feeling of support on their muscles will make the pain go away. The reason why they instinctively do that actually has nothing to do with the problem—it has to do with the fact that they haven't stretched. After all, why do people rub their back when it's sore? Because by rubbing, they are attempting to alleviate the tightness in muscles that have painfully contracted.

You might literally feel "knots" when you rub (or someone else might, if you are smart and are having someone else do the massage). Simply put, knots are muscles that haven't been stretched, so they clamp up and harden. The kneading, the pressure of the massage therapist's hands and the stretching that you feel during a properly done massage are what breaks down the knots.

Massage also helps your muscles by increasing the blood flow to them. Muscles need blood, as that's what cleans them out and replenishes them. (Remember, the discs in your spine are avascular, so they will never need a blood supply in order to function properly.) This extra blood flow is wonderfully stimulating, which is why I don't see massage therapy as a luxury, but as a necessary and helpful form of therapy that literally gets the knots out.

But if you can't afford regular massages, take heart. If you stretch your muscles on a daily basis, you should not have knots forming in the first place! You'll keep your muscles firm and pliant—and more tolerant of the stresses put on them by regular activities. And if you warm up to get your heart rate up and then do your seven stretches before you do your sport or after your workout, your more flexible muscles will make all the other exercises you do more efficient.

Can You Treat the Pain with Ice or Heat?

Patients ask me every day if they should use heat or ice on their aching back. I tell them that they should use whatever makes them feel better, because in my opinion, neither is actually necessary.

Since you now know more about inflammation, you need to revise your thinking about hurrying to get ice on your back when it starts hurting. Ice is recommended for the kind of inflammation where there is swelling in the tissues due to a traumatic event, like twisting your ankle or wrenching your knee or even cutting your finger, and for overuse injuries, like when a baseball player has a sore arm after a big game. Ice constricts; it makes muscles tighten up. For these kind of injuries, ice stops the inflammation from getting worse and reduces the blood flow to the area. This is great if you're treating a swollen or overused joint, but it is not necessarily so great if your back is sore. Remember, back inflammation is not the same as inflammation in an injured joint, as there is no fluid and there is no swelling. So all the ice will do is numb your skin.

From a logical standpoint, heat is better at loosening up and stimulating the muscles in your back that are constricting and tight. If you can pinpoint the area that hurts—and with back pain, that's not always easy—then heat might help the muscles relax a little more, and it will certainly bring additional blood flow into the area.

If you do like ice, though, it's not going to harm your back muscles, but if you're not careful, it might irreparably harm your skin by freezing it (which is akin to a burn). Never put ice directly on your skin, and try leaving it on for at least a half hour, but no more than an hour.

Pain Medications

We live in a society where many people go to the doctor when they feel bad, and either their overworked and time-pressed physician hands them a prescription just in case or they demand medication, because they'd rather take something than nothing.

I see the effects of overmedication and improper medication every single day. By the time nearly all my patients come to see me, they've likely already been to the emergency room or urgent care center, and how were they treated there? They were examined; they perhaps had an X-ray; they perhaps were given an injection of a super-potent pain medication, like Demerol or morphine, if they were in excruciating pain; and they were then given a prescription for a potent pain medication and/or some form of an anti-inflammatory medication, like Motrin, and told to see a specialist.

Here's the problem with these pain medications: their function is to help you manage pain. While they're certainly great at doing this, and can temporarily minimize or eradicate pain, they do nothing to *heal* the injury—and they don't address the primary problem, which is *what caused* the back pain! This can set you up for an endless cycle of pain and then treatment with medication and then temporary improvement and then pain again. And when pain escalates, so does the potency of the medication, which can lead to extremely serious side effects and addiction.

I don't prescribe Valium for lower back pain, but I can say that it is often prescribed, because many, many people love it. In fact, they love it so much that it's commonly referred to as vitamin V. But I think Valium is a very poor choice for people with back problems. It's an antipsychotic drug that often causes drowsiness, and it's used as a muscle relaxant because it basically relaxes everything and makes you feel like jelly.

Valium is highly addictive and causes depression, but the fact that it helps a lot of people sleep is one of the reasons it's often handed out like candy. It is an awful situation when you're in so much pain that you can't sleep. But there's a big problem to think about when you have an acute episode of low back pain and you take a knockout prescription pain pill your doctor gave you. If the only thing the pill does is knock you out, you're going to wake up with the same back pain you went to sleep with, and it might even feel worse.

The reason I don't recommend narcotics for the majority of low back pain cases is simple. It's far better to start with the least invasive treatment—namely, the stretches in this book, with perhaps an anti-inflammatory—and see what happens than go right to a narcotic, which can create an entirely unnecessary set of very difficult problems to handle.

Another important reason I steer away from narcotics is that my goal is to help you break the cycle of back pain, which is what stretching will do. But if you are prescribed heavy-duty medications, it's all too easy to start relying on the medication and not address the issue. And you do not address the issue, if you do not start a treatment plan, you can, paradoxically, end up with even more pain. If you do nothing, a muscle that is tight on Monday will be far tighter and excruciating by Friday, making you feel that you must up the dosage of the pain medication in order to cope. Then the cycle escalates from there.

Avoiding the root issue is like paying only the minimum balance on your credit card while spending the maximum. Pretty soon you'll have a big problem, and you'll spend years paying off the interest instead of the principal.

Trust me when I say that the best muscle relaxer that we have is not Valium. Instead, it is a very inexpensive, easily available over-the-counter drug that you likely already have in your medicine cabinet—ibuprofen (its brand-name counterparts include Motrin and Advil). Ibuprofen is what's called a nonsteroidal anti-inflammatory (or NSAID) medication.

NSAIDs work on back inflammation because, as you know, this is not the kind of inflammation that involves swelling and fluid. NSAIDs decrease your body's inflammatory *response*—the response that occurs when there's an injury to some part of your spine, that is, when signals are sent to your muscles, your muscles tighten up and stop working properly in order to protect your spine, and a lot of pain happens in the process.

If you have acute back pain, NSAIDs are very beneficial, especially if you take them as soon as you feel the first twinges. I think everyone with acute back pain should be on an anti-inflammatory, unless, of course, you have a contraindicating, underlying medical condition. If so, you must always check with your physician before self-medicating, even with an over-the-counter product.

The fallacy is, however, that ibuprofen is a pain medication. It's not. If you take two Advil, the pain factor might be the same twenty minutes later. For maximum effect, you need to gradually build up the dosage in a process that only your physician or orthopedist can specify.

Many athletes that I know and that I treat use ibuprofen regularly, especially before they play their sport. It's a great idea, as it is a proactive step you can take that will automatically decrease your body's inflammatory response to the normal kind of muscle use and spine movements you'll engage in whenever you work out or play a sport.

What about Pain Creams and Patches?

If you're looking for pain relief at the pharmacy, you'll find shelves laden with products claiming to be the magic pill or cream or patch to ease your woes. Do any of them really work?

There are two primary kinds of over-the-counter topical products: those that "heat" up the area and those that cool it down. The heat products are those like BENGAY or Tiger Balm, and when you apply them, you definitely feel warmth and perhaps some tingling. This is due to the active analgesic (or pain-relieving) ingredients, usually methyl salicylate and menthol, which increase blood flow where applied. The cooling products, such as lidocaine patches, are a topical anesthetic that temporarily diminishes nerve pain.

Do these products really work? Lidocaine is effective for temporarily reducing pain, but the effect lasts only for a short period of time. The heat-creating creams and lotions may help some people in large part due to the placebo effect. If you feel warmth in an area that's sore, and if you believe that it's helping, what are you going to do? You're going to relax your muscles. You will release some of the tension and fear you've been holding in, fear that if you move or breathe deeply, you might cause more damage. And the more your muscles relax, the more the pain will decrease and the sooner you can get back to normal functioning.

Feel free to use these products if you like them and if you feel that they can help you, and be sure to follow the directions. Applying more cream than indicated will not provide more pain relief. Or you can try a heating pad, as it will pretty much do the same thing.

Just remember that as with any temporary fix, these products can't address the problem that caused the pain in the first place.

How I Treat Patients Who Come to Me with Low Back Pain

There are two categories of patients who come to see me. The first is those with the typical, horribly excruciating, incredibly common lower back pain, whom this book will help. The second is those who have more serious problems, which warrant a higher level of treatment; you can read about these conditions in the Appendix. And although the pain is horrific, you want to be in the first category, because you should get better without invasive treatment.

Almost all my new patients are incredibly fearful and assume the worst, and of course, I can't blame them for that when their pain is so severe. Usually the first thing they expect me to do is take an X-ray, but this is usually unnecessary. One of the most prominent myths about typical lower back pain is that an X-ray is needed for a diagnosis, but in truth X-rays are not needed during the initial consultation unless the pain is associated with trauma or had lasted for more than six to eight weeks. X-rays do not show nerves, soft tissue or herniated discs, so for patients with sciatica, for example, an MRI would be needed.

Once I discuss the diagnosis, I assure most of my patients that they will get better within three to six weeks. Then I add that treatment of their low back pain is a process. There is no instant magic bullet or pill to take. But stretching is as close to a magic bullet as they're going to get. I also inform them that they might need a few sessions with a chiropractor or with a physical therapist, and a regular dose of an anti-inflammatory NSAID medication. But I underscore that it's the *movement* of stretching their muscles that will help them most of all. And I tell them that once they get over the current bout of back pain, continuing with the seven stretches and core strengthening is a must-do to prevent future occurrences of back pain.

Many of my patients are very surprised, if not shocked, when I explain this to them. They tell me that they can barely move now as it is, so how can stretching help them when they can't even envision how they can get down on the floor? Shouldn't they stay in bed?

I answer by explaining that bed rest for back pain, which used to be the treatment years ago, is by far the worst thing they can do. Progressive *stretching* is by far the best thing they can do for acute back pain. I then add that these stretches are very gentle and easy to do, and will relieve the tightness in their muscles that is causing the pain.

When these patients ask how long it will take for them to be out of pain, I tell them it's usually within that three-to-six-week period. That doesn't mean they're going to be in such acute pain for four to five weeks, but that if they start to incorporate these stretches into their daily routine, by week six they should be able to get back into their normal routine.

The overwhelming majority of patients with typical lower back pain who follow my instructions get better. I mean "completely out of pain" better. And if they keep stretching and strengthening their core, they will help prevent similar injuries in the future and will minimize the pain and the length of their recuperation in the future.

If, however, they are in the minority (about 10 to 15 percent of low back pain patients I see) and are diligent about stretching and take anti-inflammatory medications, like NSAIDs, yet do not get measurable relief, then we need to do more testing and explore other possibilities. They might need only an injection of steroids, along with more chiropractic and/or physical therapy treatments for a few weeks. The steroids can provide a little boost to the healing process, as they inhibit the inflammatory process, but the goal is the same—to get rid of the pain and to be capable of doing the stretches.

In the worst-case scenario, surgery might be needed. The Appendix explains why. But most of my patients who do need surgery have underlying issues that are more complicated than typical low back pain.

Dealing with the Fear of Chronic Pain

No one should have chronic back pain. No one should wake up in the morning with the first thought in their heads being how much their back hurts and the second thought being how they are going to get up and manage to make it through the day. Not in the twenty-first century, with the treatment possibilities that should be easily available to you!

It is very upsetting to me as a back surgeon whose goal is to help people lead healthy, pain-free lives that so many of my patients have given up. I can't tell you how many of them feel utterly hopeless because the pain has been there for so long and no one has been able to help them, and because the myths about low back pain are so potent. They're led to feel that, oh, well, there's nothing they can do, no one's really paying attention, and it's not their heart or lungs or cancer or a tumor or some other horrible disease that's going to kill them, so they'll just have to take some medication and deal with it.

But "dealing" with back pain is not the same as treating it to make it go away. It's a huge quality of life issue. It causes stress and depression. How can anyone not be depressed if they have to give up the activities or sports they love, or if they can't even pick up their child for a hug without twinges of terrible pain? How can anyone not be depressed if they can't sit at work and their livelihood might be at stake? How can anyone not be depressed if they fear that the pain will get worse and they might become permanently disabled?

If, on the other hand, you begin to believe that you're not a lost cause, and that your back problem and the resulting pain are so incredibly common that you can almost think of them as *normal*, you might start to have some hope. And then if I tell you that *you can overcome your pain,* you should have more than hope—you should have a new goal.

This new goal is to be proactive and fight your back pain. It is a battle you *will* win—because you've got a secret weapon on your side.

That weapon is stretching.

WHY STRETCHING IS THE KEY TO MANAGING BACK PAIN

I love to play golf, but quite some years ago I was making no progress, so I went to a highly recommended golf pro for advice and a few lessons. The first thing he asked me was, "How often do you stretch before you play?"

When I told him I didn't stretch, to his credit, he didn't roll his eyes. Instead, he said, "That's one of your biggest mistakes. If you want to change what you're doing and get better, let me tell you, every professional golfer stretches. You might not see them do it, but they stretch. Every professional football player or baseball player is out on the fields, stretching, before a game. I can't tell you how important it is to stretch your muscles. It'll prevent injuries, and it'll make your game a lot better than hitting five thousand practice balls might do."

Point taken! But, of course, stretching isn't just for professional athletes—every human body will benefit from daily stretching. It will improve not just your athletic ability. It will improve how you play the game of life.

Look at it this way: the game may be that you want to get in your car and drive to work, and be healthy enough to get through the workday without being in pain, and then drive home and have a nice dinner and a relaxing evening with your family. That's the game I want to play and that Cara wants to play, and we both take the few minutes needed every day to keep ourselves at the top of our game. Sure, we might not be stretching for the Super Bowl or the World Series, but we're stretching for our own game plan so we can function at the top of our form and do what it is we're here to do.

Stretching is incredibly effective. It can help lessen your back pain and help you avoid more problems in the future. Some form of stretching is at the top of the list of treatments I prescribe for my patients with acute back pain.

If you are in bad pain now, start these stretches slowly and gently. Not surprisingly, though, it is best to learn how to stretch when you aren't in pain. That way, you can go through the entire motion without worrying if it will cause more pain, and you will develop muscle strength and flexibility, which will lessen both the severity and duration of any back pain you endure in the future.

Stretching Does a Body Good

- It improves blood circulation to the muscles and joints
- It makes you more flexible
- It improves your posture
- It helps relieve stress
- It helps with your coordination
- It reduces muscle soreness and tension
- It gives you greater body awareness and mental alertness
- You can do it anywhere, anytime

- You don't need to be an athlete to do it
- You don't need to be exercising regularly to do it
- It doesn't matter how old (or young) you are—you can still stretch
- You don't need to buy anything to do it
- There is no downside
- It helps you get rid of your lower back pain

Stretching and Your Muscles

As you read in the first section of this chapter, strengthening the muscles that support the spine is one of the most important components in the treatment and prevention of low back pain.

Stretching is what happens when a specific skeletal muscle or muscle group is deliberately elongated, often by abduction (movement away from the axis of your body), in order to improve the muscle's elasticity and flexibility.

Muscles are made up of fibers. Like all fibers and other components of your body, they need nutrients. They also need to be constantly stimulated. The more you stimulate your muscles, the more you build up fibers that are strong and flexible; the more you don't stimulate your muscles, the more they weaken, as their fibers lose strength and responsiveness.

Without regular stimulation, the muscle fibers that you need to lift objects, stand up straight, walk, run and build endurance won't be there when you need them. Trying to use muscles that lack strength can cause injuries—it's one of the reasons why shoveling snow is responsible for so many back problems. And you may be horrified to find out that muscles that aren't stimulated are replaced with fat. Not the healthy fat that we need for optimal brain functioning and that keeps our skin supple, but the kind of fat that is thick, viscous and clogging.

All muscle fibers require oxygenation, or oxygen in order to function properly. Oxygen is to muscles what gas is to your car. Some muscle fibers are aerobic fibers. Other muscle fibers are anaerobic, which means they need a lot less oxygen to work properly. Aerobic fibers are particularly needed for endurance. For example, marathon runners build up a huge amount of aerobic fibers in their muscles because they run for a long period of time, so oxygen must keep stimulating and replenishing their leg muscles to keep them pumping. Weight lifters and sprinters, on the other hand, are more in need of anaerobic fibers, because they don't need constant regeneration. If you're only going to lift weights in a competition or run fifty or one hundred yards at blazing speeds, once the muscle fibers serve their function, they don't need to be replenished; they can simply burn off. This is why sprinters have such immense muscles full of anaerobic fibers, which means their muscle mass is larger, whereas distance runners have long and lean aerobic fibers.

Ideally, you want to have a good ratio of anaerobic and aerobic fibers in your muscles. Since stretching stimulates muscles, it allows these fibers to attain and remain in a healthy balance. Without this, you can build up a lot of caustic lactic acid, which causes soreness and pain.

Don't think that healthy muscle fibers are needed just by sprinters or endurance runners. Even if you're used to doing just a half hour of fitness walking every day (or you are a couch potato), you can't strengthen your muscles well unless you stretch them. It's the stretching that gives muscles the limber suppleness they need. A muscle that is rigid, tight and contracted is a muscle whose fibers are not functioning properly. It'll be so seized up that it becomes too painful to move.

Think of your muscles as toddlers. They have a very short attention span. They need to be built up slowly. Doubtless you know that if you try and push yourself at some exercise or sport—running for two miles when you've never even run a half mile before, or hitting the gym with the firm resolve to get in shape, and working out on the weight machines for an hour during your first session—you will pay later that night or certainly the next day, when your muscles are practically groaning in agony. What you want to do is start small and gradually increase both the duration and intensity of the activity. This will not only strengthen your muscles but also prevent injuries and burnout.

For instance, perhaps the first time you work out with weights, you lift for twenty minutes and feel incredibly sore and burnt out the next day, but after three months of regular sessions two or three times a week, you're up to forty-five minutes without any pain the next day.

After a year, you're up to over an hour, and you feel pretty great after each session. There's no pain, soreness or stiffness.

Why Stretching Certain Muscles Is So Important

Why do we stretch the particular muscles you'll read all about in Chapter 2, and not other muscles? Why will you be stretching your quadriceps and hamstrings, found in the front and back of your thighs, or your piriformis muscles, located at the back of your hips, and not your shoulder muscles?

The reason is simple: all the muscles you'll engage in the seven stretches are attached to a central point—namely, your pelvis. And the muscles attached to your pelvis are what stabilize your spine. Each one of these muscles has a role in pulling on your pelvis and lower back, causing strain and sometimes pulling you out of the ideal neutral spine position.

You already learned on p.19 that the muscles in your body play agonist/antagonist roles; they are meant to work together for maximum power. If one muscle is not functioning correctly, is injured or is atrophied, it will affect the function of the muscle it works with synergistically. Stretching the major muscles attached to the pelvis/spine works them as a whole. This makes the muscles less likely to seize up and cause you pain.

Like anything else in life, the more time you put into stretching your muscles, the better the results.

Stretching Also Improves Flexibility

Flexibility is your joint's ability to move through a full range of motion. Stretching prevents tightness and stiff muscles, which can restrict our daily physical activities and put us at greater risk of injury. Better flexibility maximizes balance, coordination and mobility, which means less likelihood of falling. This is especially important because as our bodies get older, our joints naturally become stiffer and tighter, so stretching is the ideal way to loosen them up.

CHAPTER 2

THE BASICS OF STRETCHING, PROTECTION MODE AND HOW TO MOVE WHEN YOU'RE IN PAIN

THE SEVEN BASIC STRETCHES

These simple stretches are the heart of this book. Once you do all seven and see how great each stretch and core routine makes you feel, you will never forget them. Not only will you help yourself get out of pain, but you will also strengthen your body and improve your overall health and fitness.

Before You Start

Once your back-strengthening and stretching routine is a regular part of your daily life, doing these steps will be as natural and easy to you as breathing.

What to Wear

Your clothing should be loose and comfortable. For example, you can do your stretching in pajamas or yoga clothes. Avoid jeans or any kind of tighter-fitting clothing, as they can constrict movement and dig into your skin. You can wear socks, but not if you're stretching on a floor where you can slip, either go barefoot or wear socks and lightweight athletic shoes.

Where to Do It

Try to do your stretches on a non-slippery surface, like a rug or carpet. It is worth investing in a yoga or exercise mat with a nonslip backing, as they are very inexpensive and will last for years. The extra bit of cushioning makes a difference, and you can place the mat anywhere.

Stay Hydrated

Although stretches are not aerobic exercises, you still need to drink water throughout the day to stay hydrated.

Always Warm Up Before Stretching

Even though this stretching sequence is very short, it is extremely important to do these stretches after a short warm-up, if at all possible. The reason for a warm-up is to get the blood and oxygen flowing to your muscles to prevent injuries. If your muscles are "cold," you might inadvertently cause damage to them, leading to muscle soreness and downtime, which you certainly don't want to have.

- This warm-up only has to take 5 to 10 minutes and should consist of some sort of easy to moderate cardiovascular activity.

- If your back pain is manageable and you can walk, that's what you should do—walk! Have a short walk around the house, or if you have an elliptical machine or a treadmill, walk on that with no incline. If you are up to it and have your doctor's permission, you can also slowly jog in place for a few minutes. Jogging outside is even better (count that as your aerobic exercise of the day, which is good for everybody capable of doing it), if the weather and your schedule permit.

- If it hurts even to walk around the house, or if it's more comfortable, seated jogging is an option. You can do this while sitting in a supportive yet firm chair, on an exercise ball or on the edge of a bed. Seated jogging is jogging in place while seated, pumping your opposite arms and legs at the same time while engaging your core to keep you balanced.

- A standing wall jog is another alternative. Place an exercise ball between your back and the wall for support; then lean back against it while pumping your opposite arms and legs at the same time. This will raise your heart rate without aggravating your back.

- If you don't have time or your back is hurting, you can take a warm shower.

- If you don't feel comfortable doing any of the above, wait at least ten minutes after you get out of bed to begin your stretches.

- If you're in so much pain that you can't get out of bed, your primary goal should only be to get up and lessen the pain. Anything you can do to increase your range of motion will help ease the back pain.

Concentrate on Your Form

Both Cara and I have often seen people at the gym whose form is so off base that what they're doing is counterproductive—and sometimes even puts them at risk for injuries. It is much better to start slow and take your time with all these movements until you've memorized them. This way you'll work your muscles perfectly.

- Be sure to follow all the instructions exactly. For instance, it is extremely important to know how to contract your abdominals correctly. (Need I say that one of the most gratifying side benefits is a much more toned belly!)

- Never bounce during a stretch. Move slowly and steadily.

- Do not go for the burn! You should feel tension in the muscles, *not* pain.

- Just breathe naturally, in a way that makes you feel calm and comfortable. Be sure to never, ever hold your breath while stretching.

How Do You Know How Far to Stretch?

When done properly, stretching can feel really good. A gentle pull or tension is the essence of the stretch, which is why "feel the burn" is a phrase we wish people would forget. It creates a mind-set that views stretching as some sort of competitive sport, when that's the last thing it should be.

Bear in mind that since no two bodies are alike, your ability to stretch is not going to be the same as anyone else's. Just as it might be frustratingly true that you can work out as hard as the next person yet not achieve the same muscle growth, you can try to stretch and might find you don't have the same flexibility as the person next to you in yoga class, too. Because some people may not be able to stretch their muscles as far, or they might not feel the same amount of tension as others do when they stretch the same way, we've provided alternatives and modifications to the stretches. If you're a beginner, you'll be using your muscles in a new way, so don't push past your comfort zone. The more you stretch, the more you will be able to stretch. Do not push your limbs beyond the angles shown in these photographs.

What you want to avoid is stretching to the point where you feel pain. If there are any twinges in your back from the stretch itself, stop immediately, as you might have gone too far. Ease back to where you don't feel any pain; then hold the stretch at that point.

Since stretching should never hurt, if you feel any discomfort that is not your typical back pain, slow down, as you might be overdoing it. If you are afraid you'll hurt your back, then contract your abdominals and find a comfortable position. Start stretching again when you feel more confident.

How to Breathe Properly

Here's an easy way to ensure that you are breathing properly. Watch how babies breathe and you'll see how it's done!

❶ Lie on your back, knees bent, feet flat on the floor.

❷ Place your hands on the lower part of your stomach, then breathe in (inhale) slowly through your nose and breathe out (exhale) through your mouth. The movement should come from your belly, and your hands should move up and down.

How to Do an Abdominal Contraction

This is one of the most important sections in the book, although it might seem a bit silly and like something you already know how to do. All you have to do is suck it in, right? On the contrary. In fact, we've found that few people, including professional athletes, have been taught how to do an abdominal contraction that creates a stiffness to brace the spine.

Your abdominals are like a girdle for your back; they stabilize and protect your spine, and when you contract them you will also feel your back muscles contract. You will then contract your pelvic floor muscles. This should feel like a tightness around your stomach and back (your core). With this strong brace you have activated, you can strengthen your back without injury.

The Abdominal Contraction

To tighten and brace your spine:

❶ First lie on your back with your knees bent, feet flat on the floor. Breathe in through your nose and out through your mouth and relax. Place your hands loosely on your pelvic area, right above your genitals, and cough. Do you feel that area moving slightly up and down, with a slight tension? That is your transverse abdominal muscle.

❷ Next, inhale, and on your exhale, draw in your belly toward your spine to create stiffness. You should also feel your low back muscles tightening. Hold the contraction for a few seconds and then release it. It should feel like a corset tightening up around you.

❸ In the same position, place your hands on your pelvis to feel the contraction; pretend you have to urinate and contract your muscles to stop the flow, or you have a bowel movement and you have to hold it in. This is a Kegel exercise, used to contract your pelvic floor muscles.

4 Now that you get the picture, let's put it together.

5 Place your hands back on your pelvic area. Inhale, and on the exhale, pull your belly toward your spine to tighten. As you contract, you will be pulling your belly away from your hands and you should also feel the contraction in your back. Then do a Kegel exercise.

6 This is a tightening feeling, not a feeling like you are sucking in your stomach. Your stomach should not protrude at all during this contraction. You must always breathe, so don't hold your breath.

7 Practice the abdominal contraction as much as you can so it becomes second nature. Do it very carefully and gently, and don't force anything. Do them while waiting for an elevator or while stuck in line at the grocery store, and you won't feel like you're totally wasting your time. Try to focus on your breathing, as doing the contractions on the exhale is not as simple as it seems at first. The more you make these contractions a regular part of your life, the more protected your back will be when you're going about your daily routine.

How to Get on the Floor or Lower Yourself When Stretching

1 Contracting your abdominals throughout the movement, slowly get down on the floor. Use your hands or whatever support you need to lower yourself.

2 Once you're on the floor, place your feet in front of you and your elbows behind you, then slowly lie down with your knees bent.

SEVEN STRETCHES/ SEVEN MINUTES

Ideally, you should do these stretches two to three times daily when you're in a cycle of pain, and then once a day or more, depending on your lifestyle (if, for example, you have to sit at work for long periods, you may only be able to do these stretches once daily). They take only seven minutes to do. They're especially helpful if done right before bed. If you straighten up the house or take the dog for a short walk right before you stretch, not only will you be productive, but you'll also warm your body up without thinking about it (and your dog will be happy!).

THE 7 STRETCHES	MUSCLE AREA WORKED
1. Hamstring Wall or Floor Stretch	Back of thighs
2. Knees to Chest Stretch	Hips / Buttocks / Lower back
3. Spinal Stretch	Lower back / Sides of lower back
4. Piriformis Stretch	Buttocks
5. Hip Flexors Stretch	Hips / Front of thighs
6. Quadriceps Standing or Lying-Down Stretch	Front of thighs
7. Total Back Stretch	Entire back / Shoulders / Arms

Before You Start: The Abdominal Contraction

WHAT IT DOES: Supports and helps to protect your back

This is one of our secret weapons for protecting your back. It can be done whenever you like throughout the day from a standing, sitting or lying position. This contraction trains your abdominals so they can brace your spine with every movement to prevent injury.

1 If you are on the floor or in bed, make sure you are lying on your back. Bend your knees and place your arms at your sides.

2 Inhale, and then, on the exhale, slowly contract your abdominals.

3 Hold this position for five to ten seconds, but do not hold your breath.

4 Do this ten times.

5 If you are standing, start at Step 2.

1a. Hamstring Wall Stretch

WHAT IT DOES: Stretches the back of your thighs

1 Contract your abdominals, get down on the floor, and lie faceup near a protruding corner of a room or near a door frame.

2 Place the heel of your left foot up against the wall and bring your buttocks up so that they touch the wall or get as close to it as possible. Slide your left leg up the wall until it is straight or slightly bent. Slide your right leg forward on the floor until it is straight or slightly bent.

3 Hold this position for thirty seconds. You will feel a stretch in the back of your leg. Try to keep both hips flat on the floor.

4 Slowly slide your left leg down on the wall until your left knee bends. Then bring your right leg into a bent-knee position. Contract your abdominals; then turn your body to the side, assuming a fetal position, so you can get up. Repeat this stretch, with the right leg doing what the left leg did.

5 Do this two times for each leg.

If you do this stretch in a doorway, make sure it is wide enough. Do this stretch only if you feel comfortable using the wall as an anchor. This technique is much safer for your back than standing and bending forward when doing a hamstring stretch.

1b. Hamstring Floor Stretch — Variation 1

1 Lie on your back on the floor, knees bent. Place your hands or a belt, band or towel behind your calf, thigh or foot, whichever makes you feel most comfortable and allows you to feel the most tension in your hamstring, and slowly raise your right leg and straighten it as much as you can, until you feel the stretch in the back of your leg. You can keep your leg slightly bent if you need to.

2 Try to straighten your left leg. If you feel any tension in your back, leave your left leg bent.

3 Hold this position for thirty seconds.

4 Bend your left leg to a bent-knee position; then bring your right leg down to a bent knee. Repeat this stretch by raising your left leg instead of your right.

5 Do this two times with each leg.

When switching legs or at anytime during this stretch, do not place both legs straight out on the floor.

Contract your abdominals when bringing your legs up.

2. Knees to Chest Stretch

WHAT IT DOES: Stretches your hips, buttocks and lower back

1 Lie on your back, knees bent, feet flat on the floor, arms at your sides. Contract your abdominals, and using your hands, bring your right knee up toward your chest.

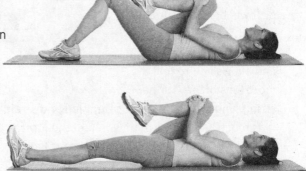

2 With your abdominals contracted, try to straighten your left leg. If you feel any tension in your back, leave your left leg bent.

3 Hold this position for twenty seconds.

4 Before you bring your right knee down from the stretch, make sure to bend your left knee. Then repeat the stretch, bring your left knee up toward your chest.

5 With your abdominals contracted, from the starting position, bring your right knee up and then your left knee up, and hold for ten seconds.

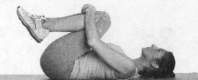

6 Bring one leg down at a time.

3a. Spinal Stretch

WHAT IT DOES: Stretches your lower back and the sides of your lower back

1 Lie on your back, knees bent, feet flat on the floor, arms out at your sides.

2 Contract your abdominals, and then pull your right knee to your chest with both hands and straighten your left leg out on the floor.

3 Place your right arm straight out on your right side, keeping your abdominals contracted. Then, with your left hand, slowly bring your right knee over toward your left side.

4 Keep your left hand on your right knee, with your right foot resting on the back of your left knee, and turn your head toward your right side.

5 Hold the stretch for twenty seconds. Do not force your right knee to the floor, and make sure your head, arms and shoulders stay on the floor. Try not to arch your back.

6 With your abdominals contracted, slowly return both knees to a bent position.

7 Repeat the stretch with your left knee.

Make sure your abdominals are contracted when bringing your knees up and over.

3b. Spinal Stretch—Variation 1

❶ Lie on your back, knees
bent, feet flat on the floor,
arms at your sides.

❷ Contract your abdominals, and bring both
knees to your left side.

❸ Hold the stretch for
twenty seconds. Then, with your abdominals contracted, slowly
bring your knees back to the starting position.

❹ Repeat the stretch, bringing both knees to your right side.

*Make sure you keep your abdominals contracted when bringing your knees
to one side or the other, and keep your head and arms down.*

4a. Piriformis Stretch

WHAT IT DOES: Stretches your buttocks

❶ Lie on your back, knees bent, feet
flat on the floor, arms at
your sides.

❷ Contract your abdominals, and cross your right leg over
your left, resting your right foot
on your left knee.

❸ With your abdominals contracted, grab
your left thigh with both
hands and bring both legs
toward your body.

④ Hold this position for thirty seconds.

⑤ With your abdominals contracted, bring both legs down to a bent-knee position, and repeat the stretch with your left leg.

4b. Piriformis Stretch — Variation 1

① Lie on your back, knees bent, arms at your side.

② Contract your abdominals, and cross your right leg over your left, resting your right foot on your left knee, then raise your left leg, keeping your left knee bent.

③ Push down with your right leg, and push up with your left leg.

④ Hold this position for thirty seconds. Slowly bring your knees back to the starting position.

⑤ Cross your left leg over your right leg, and repeat the stretch.

5a. Hip Flexors Stretch

WHAT IT DOES: Stretches your hips and the front of your thighs

① Contract your abdominals, and kneel down, placing your right foot behind you and your left leg in a bent-knee position with your left foot flat on the floor. If you have knee problems, put a pillow under your right knee.

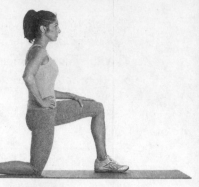

② Place your right hand on your waist and your left hand gently on your left leg for support. If you're worried about balance, hold on to a sturdy chair placed at your left side.

③ With your abdominals contracted, lean forward into your right hip while keeping the right knee on the floor. You will feel the stretch in the front of your right hip.

④ Hold this position for thirty seconds.

⑤ Switch sides and repeat the stretch.

Make sure your abdominal muscles are contracted, your shoulders are down and your back is straight. Don't arch your back.

5b. Hip Flexor One Cheek on Chair — Variation 1

① Stand with a sturdy chair on your left side. Contract your abdominals and place only your left buttock on the seat. Keep your left leg bent in front of you. Hold on to the back of the chair with your left hand.

② Place your right leg behind you, with your toes facing forward and your heel up, so that you feel the stretch in the front of your right hip.

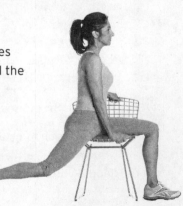

③ Hold this position for thirty seconds.

④ Switch sides and repeat the stretch.

6a. Quadriceps Standing Stretch

WHAT IT DOES: Stretches the front of your thighs

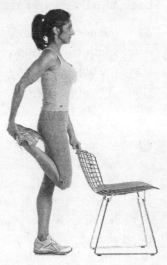

1 Stand next to a sturdy piece of furniture and hold on to it for balance with your left hand.

2 Contract your abdominals, grasp your right foot (or ankle, if that's easier) with your right hand, and gently pull your right leg back and up, with your toes pointing toward your head. Make sure your right knee remains close to your left leg. It should not move out toward your right side.

3 Hold this position for thirty seconds.

4 Switch to your left leg and repeat the stretch.

6b. Quadriceps Lying-Down Stretch — Variation 1

1 Lie on your left side. You can place a pillow under your head if you like.

2 Contract your abdominals and grasp the top of your right foot or ankle with your right hand and gently pull your heel toward your buttocks.

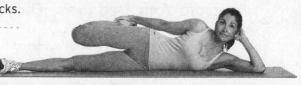

3 Hold this position for thirty seconds.

4 With your abdominals contracted, assume the fetal position, roll over onto your back and lie with your knees bent, feet flat on the floor.

5 Switch to your right side and repeat the stretch.

7. Total Back Stretch

WHAT IT DOES: Stretches your
back, shoulders and arms

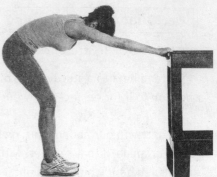

1 Stand next to a sturdy object, knees
bent. Contract your abdominals, and
grasp the object with both hands, keeping
your arms straight. Keep your head level
with your shoulders.

2 Hold this position for ten seconds.

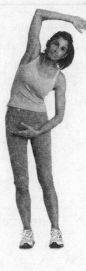

3 Stand up straight, place your left hand in front of
your body, contract your abdominals and bring your
right arm up over your head, with your elbow bent.
Bend your upper body gently to the left. You can
use the object for support if you need to.

4 Hold this position for ten seconds.

5 Repeat this stretch, bringing your left arm up
over your head.

Variation: Stretches and Exercises to Do from Your Bed (Yes, They Really Work!)

For those with back pain who have a hard time even getting out of bed
in the morning, we have devised an effective sequence of stretches and
exercises that can be done in bed. See Chapter 5 for more details.

Cara's Personal Stretching Routine

Once you learn how to do the stretches, try my routine. I do one side at a time, then alternate.

A. Right Side

1. Hamstring Floor Stretch	30-60 seconds
2. Knees to Chest Stretch	20 seconds
3. Spinal Stretch	20 seconds

B. Left Side

1. Hamstring Floor Stretch	30-60 seconds
2. Knees to Chest Stretch	20 seconds
3. Spinal Stretch	20 seconds

C. Both Sides

1. Knees to Chest Stretch	10 seconds
2. Piriformis Stretch on the right side	30 seconds
Piriformis Stretch on the left side	30 seconds
3. Hip Flexors Stretch on the right side	30 seconds
Hip Flexors Stretch on the left side	30 seconds
4. Quadriceps Standing on the right side	30 seconds
Quadriceps Standing on the left side	30 seconds
5. Total Back Stretch	30 seconds

Can I Do These Stretches Even If I'm in Acute Pain?

Yes, you can!

One of the most important points in this book is that the specific muscles related to lower back pain have to be stretched daily. But even if you get to the point where you are stretching every day and have completely alleviated your back pain, you also know by now that back pain can show up again for no reason whatsoever. If that happens, you do not have to panic—because you know that these stretches *will always work*, so you can manage your pain.

Here are a few tips about doing these stretches when you're in pain:

- If the pain comes on when you awaken in the morning, try to warm up your body with careful movement, such as walking around your house, walking outside on a level surface or walking in place, as you know by now how important it is to not stretch cold muscles. If, however, this episode of pain comes on during the day or at night, you should be warmed up already from daily activity, so it's okay to start stretching without worrying about a warm-up.

- If any careful movement is too painful, you should wait at least five to ten minutes before beginning the seven stretches.

- As hard as it can be, try to relax and remember to breathe normally when stretching. Clenching all your muscles from tension and worry can make the pain worse.

- If you feel that you are not ready to stretch, try using ice for 15-20 minutes prior to stretching. Always wait at least an hour between each icing period.

- Try to get up and walk around, if possible, if you are not ready to stretch.

PROTECTION MODE
How to Move and What to Do
When Back Pain Hits

No matter where you are when your back goes out and the pain comes on—usually without any warning—you *can* get to a safe position. This is one of the most important points you will learn in this book. You will use Protection Mode, and it will not let you down!

Protection Mode is a safe position that neutralizes the stress on your spine. It is based on contracting and tightening your abdominal, pelvic floor and lower back muscles; these contractions are what brace and support your back. You also pivot your feet, enabling you to turn your body as a whole, instead of having the turn come from your back only. Protection Mode thus allows you to move wherever you need to with greater confidence.

Protection Mode is as much psychological as it is physical. As discussed in Chapter 1, I know that the fear of moving and thus causing further harm can almost be as bad as the pain itself. Protection Mode, on the other hand, will always work for you, because it enables you to move. It also will prove to you that you do not have to be afraid to move. If you know that you can get into a safe position that will not harm your back, the fear and worry should automatically lessen. Cara has lived through this, as when her back used to seize up, she literally could not move either of her feet for fear of the pain and of inadvertently worsening her condition. She would look around in a panic and become stuck in one position. She felt as if she had no control over what was happening to her body, which caused her to tense up even more. When this happened when she was alone in her home, it was a very scary place to be. She knew deep down that she would *not* cause further harm to her back if she moved, and she would *not* become paralyzed, but the fear took over, anyway. Now that she has Protection Mode, however, that fear is long gone.

You might want to memorize these Protection Mode basics, so you can recite them to yourself when you need them most. They walk you through what to do so you can manage any back pain situation.

THE BASICS OF PROTECTION MODE ARE:

❶ Contract your abdominal muscles.

❷ Try to relax. We know that when you're alone and back pain strikes, you can easily start to panic. Don't give in to the fear. You can do it. You are already in pain, so it really can't get worse!

❸ Breathe normally. Do not hold your breath—that creates more tension and your whole body becomes clenched.

❹ Do not be afraid to move. You will not hurt your back any further.

❺ If you have to turn your body to move in any direction, pivot one foot at a time, and then turn your other foot and the rest of your body as a whole. Do not initiate the turn from your back. Use a sturdy object for support, if possible.

Using Protection Mode if You Are Standing

❶ Contract your abdominals, and keep breathing normally. Do *not* hold your breath!

❷ Use your feet to guide you. Slowly turn your foot that is closest to a sturdy object, and start to move as slowly and gently toward the object as possible.

❸ Turn like this: pivot one foot first, and then slowly turn your other foot and your body as one. Do not initiate this turning with your back.

❹ When you start to move, think baby steps or little slides. Feel free to move very slowly and with tiny steps or shuffles until you are comfortable enough to pick your feet up and walk.

❺ Keep your abdominals contracted when you are moving. Keep breathing naturally.

❻ Move very slowly. You'll look and feel as if you're moving in slow motion, which is just what you need to do, as back pain can be such a shock to the system that you feel that literally you can't move. As long as you know you can use your feet to gently go wherever you need to go (to a telephone, a chair, the bed, the bathroom), you don't have to panic.

Remember, when severe pain hits, your body expends a tremendous amount of energy to help you manage it, so even the smallest movement you've done countless times in your life without a thought can be difficult to manage, as well as extremely exhausting. Move as slowly as you need to!

What Do You Do When You're Standing at Home and Back Pain Suddenly Hits?

One of Cara's worst fears was an episode of back pain hitting when she was home alone. Many of my patients are absolutely terrified they will be incapacitated, and this fear automatically makes you tense up when pain hits. This can make matters much worse, because if you're tense, you will likely forget to breathe deeply and to contract your abdominals.

As long as you have a plan, and *you know you can move and you will not further hurt your back,* you do not have to be afraid when pain hits. You will control the pain, instead of the pain controlling you.

❶ Follow the steps above, and try to get to a sturdy object with which you can brace yourself.

❷ If you are alone and cannot get to a sturdy object—*and* you are fearful that you might not be able to stay upright—contract your abdominals, place your hands on your thighs and slowly lower yourself down onto either a chair or the floor.

❸ If you prefer to lie down, always keep your knees bent. Try to support them with pillows or something sturdy, such as books. If it's too hard to keep both knees bent, depending on your comfort level at this point, keep one leg straight and the other bent. Straightening both legs will cause more strain on your back.

What Do You Do When You're Standing While Out in Public and Back Pain Suddenly Hits?

Let's say you're waiting for the elevator and all of a sudden you get that dreaded twinge. What should you do?

❶ Immediately go into Protection Mode. Contract your abdominals. Remember to breathe. Do not hold your breath.

❷ Depending on the situation, try to move toward something sturdy so you can brace yourself and not worry about falling over. Use your feet to pivot in slow motion until you can work yourself over to a wall or sturdy object.

❸ Once you get your bearings, you can figure out what to do next. You might want to call for help, or perhaps the pain will lessen and you can get to your destination. Move as slowly as you need to.

❹ If this happens when you are at the office, follow the steps for What Do You Do When You're Standing at Home and Back Pain Suddenly Hits? and try to get to the nearest chair.

Using Protection Mode if You Are Seated

Back pain that strikes when you are seated is usually a little less frightening, as you are already braced against an object and don't have to worry about falling or turning. But you still have to get up at some point!

Cara was once seated on a chair when her back went into spasms, and her husband ran in to help her get up. When he tried to pull her, the intensity of the pain left her literally seeing stars. So we devised this sequence so you can feel confident about your ability to lift yourself up when back pain hits.

❶ Contract your abdominals, and make sure you're breathing normally.

❷ If your seat has armrests, place your hands on them, lean forward slightly, bend your knees and slowly rise up. Do not hold your breath.

❸ If there are no armrests, place your hands on the seat itself, lean forward slightly, bend your knees and slowly rise up.

Using Protection Mode if You Are in Bed

Many back-pain sufferers feel that it's very important to be able to get up. If so, you will feel better knowing that you can. You may need to get to a phone within arm's reach, and at some point you will certainly need to use the bathroom and get something to eat and drink in the kitchen. Remember: if your pain is debilitating, you must call your physician, who will advise you to either come to the office to get assessed or go to a hospital. Do not self-diagnose! Use this technique to get up.

 Never be too scared to get up. Immediately go into Protection Mode.

❷ If you are on your back, contract your abdominals, and bend your knees.

❸ Slowly roll your upper body and bent knees to one side, and use your hands to assist you in getting up to a seated position.

❹ If you are already on your side, use your hands to gently push yourself up to a seated position.

❺ If you are on your stomach, try to turn onto your side slowly. If it hurts too much, use your hands to push yourself up onto your hands and knees. Remember to keep your abdominals contracted and to breathe normally the entire time.

Using Protection Mode if You Are on the Floor

Many of my patients have told me of their terror when their back seizes up when they're on the floor. Sometimes they've lain down when the pain hits, but then they're afraid to get back up. Follow these steps and move slowly. This technique always works.

❶ With your back on the floor, your knees bent, contract your abdominals while breathing, and then bring your knees together, slowly turn your lower body and your upper body at the same time, and assume the fetal position.

 Contract your abdominals and use your hands to gently push yourself up to a seated position. If the seated position feels uncomfortable, slowly get on your hands and knees, and then push yourself up gently until you are back on your feet and in a standing position.

 If you need assistance, try to move close to something sturdy and lean on or hold on to it as you try to get up.

What to Do if Back Pain Hits When You Are Bending Over

It's very common for a sudden twinge of back pain to hit when you're leaning over to pick something up, and it can be frustrating if you are in an awkward position. Follow this technique to regain an upright position.

1. Contract your abdominals and breathe normally.
2. If you're not near a sturdy object, you'll need to use your legs and body as an anchor. Bend your knees slightly.
3. Place your hands on your thighs, and press down gently. Slowly move your hands up your thighs to help you as you rise to an upright position.

Lift It Right

There is a right way and a wrong way to lift anything. Unfortunately, we've all picked things up the wrong way at some point, and some of us have paid for it!

The very worst way to lift anything is by bending over at a ninety-degree angle from your waist, with your legs straight. When you straighten up, all the force of lifting is vectored right to your lower back.

I tell all my patients, even those who are postoperative, that lifting is okay as long as they disperse the weight throughout *all* the muscles of the body. The key to doing this is to bend your knees, contract your abdominals and then lift the object as close to your body as possible. When you lift like this, the negative forces are dispersed, and not focused right at ground zero—your lower back.

Remember to keep breathing normally. It's easy to forget and to hold your breath when lifting. Here are more specific instructions:

1. Get close to the object before you lift it. Place your feet shoulder-width apart, and make sure you have a firm footing.
2. Contract your abdominals, and keep them contracted the entire time, while breathing normally.

3. Slowly bend your knees and squat down. Try to have the object between your legs, if possible, so you don't have far to reach.

4. Slowly lift the object up. Do not drop your head; keep your eyes focused forward. Do your best not to make any jerking movements when you're lifting. Bring the object up to your waist, keeping it as close to your body as possible; then slowly rise up.

The Golfer's Lift for Small, Light Objects

Lift small, light objects the same way that back-savvy golfers pick up golf balls on the green.

1. You need something sturdy for support. Golfers lean on their clubs, but if you're at home, you can use a chair, desk, cane, bed or anything that is sturdy enough to hold your body weight.

2. Get close to the object, contract your abdominals and breathe. Place one of your hands on the object used for support.

3. Lift your opposite leg up so that it points straight back while you bend at the hip of the standing leg with your knee slightly bent, and then bend forward to pick up the object. Your back will be straight when bending over.

How to Use the Stairs When Your Back Hurts

Stairs are tricky to negotiate when your back is hurting, but it's often impossible to avoid them. The key to managing them is to walk like a toddler, one step at a time. This will make going downstairs, which is often scarier than going up, less of an ordeal. Go as slowly as you need to. Use objects in your surroundings—the steps, the railings and even your body—for support. Once you are able to do this, it will release you from the fear that you can't manage stairs.

If the pain is in the center of your back, grasp the railing with the hand of your dominant side, as you will naturally have stronger muscles there.

TIP: Whether your back is hurting or not, you need to know about stair safety. Before using stairs, make sure that the railing is secure, and that there is either firm carpeting or some sort of nonslip tread on bare wood stairs.

Going Upstairs

❶ Contract your abdominals, and keep breathing naturally.

❷ Place one hand on the railing to help guide you up.

❸ Move very slowly, bringing the leg of your unaffected side up the next step, then bring the other leg to meet it on the same step.

Going Downstairs

❶ Contract your abdominals, and keep breathing naturally.

❷ Place one hand on the railing to help guide you down.

❸ Move very slowly, bringing the leg of your affected side down to the step, then bring the other leg to meet it on the same step.

Cara's Story: Steve and the Stairs

My friend Steve is a thirty-five-year-old physician well-known for his calm and compassionate bedside manner. He is a long-distance runner, but he doesn't stretch or weight train, so while he has long and lean muscles in his legs, he has no core or upper-body strength.

One night I got a panicked call from him, begging me to come over. He'd hurt his back when on an out-of-town trip, and the pain was so intense that paramedics had been called. At the hospital he was given the potent painkillers hydrocodone/codeine and then was sent home, still scared. He'd never had such searing pain in his life. The medications helped, but a few nights later, he was again in agony and in full-blown panic mode.

When I arrived at his house, Steve was frozen at the top of the stairs, his hands cupped tight around the top of the banister. "Don't touch me," he said between gritted teeth. I told him I wouldn't, but that he had to listen to me, even if what I was going to tell him didn't make sense. I then added with a smile, "I know how bad the pain is because I've lived through many similar episodes. It's my life and I know how to cope. Besides, looking at you right now reminds me of me taking care of myself when my back has seized up."

He barely managed a smile as I climbed the stairs to stand next to him. "Okay, all I'm going to do is get you away from the stairs," I said calmly. "Fair enough? You need to move, to get away from the stairs, so I can help you."

He nodded, and I said, "Do you know what it feels like to contract your abdominals? Just pretend that I'm about to punch you in the stomach. You'd tighten up, right? So what I want you to do is inhale. Then, on your exhale, pull in your belly. Okay? So now I need to touch your stomach to make sure you're contracting your abdominals while you breathe and talk to me."

Since he was able to do that, I went on. "Don't flinch, because that will hurt your back. I'm going to touch you gently with one finger." When I did, I could feel him trembling, as he was so terrified. I could also see that he was stuck behind the banister, so he couldn't back up or move forward. He was going to have to pivot to turn his body.

"Now, as long as your abs are contracted, you have created an internal brace for your spine, so when I ask you to move, I promise you it will not put any further strain on your back," I told him. "So go ahead and raise the toes of your left foot no more than two inches up. Then pivot that foot very slowly to the left. I know you're exhausted and scared. That's okay. Pivot a tiny bit, and then rest."

Once he was able to pivot into a turn, he could move away from the stairs and walk. I asked him if the pain was worse and he said no. "Good," I said. "Now we're going to inch you down to your bedroom and reassess the situation. Trust me. We're going to go as slow as possible. Rest, breathe, inhale, and then, on the exhale, contract your abdominals. I'm going to hold my hands out to you, so hold on to them as I move backward and slowly slide your feet toward me." I realized he needed to slide, as he was literally too scared to pick up his feet, but I assured him that if his abdominals were contracted, he would have more control of his back and would be able to move with-out causing further pain. Once he felt comfortable enough to move and realized he was halfway down the hall, he then tried to pick up his feet so he could walk the rest of the way.

Make sure you take your time. In the end, it took me ten minutes to walk Steve down the hall—what should normally take five seconds.

I told Steve's wife to arrange stacks of pillows on his bed and place a yoga mat on the floor. I showed him how to bend his knees so he was in a semi-squatting position, and how to slide his hands down his thighs so he could get down onto his hands and knees on the mat, before lower-ing himself all the way down and curling into a fetal position. If possible, when you're alone, this is the position you want to get into, so you can do your stretches on a flat surface.

"This is harder than running a marathon," Steve said when he was finally down on the floor and able to roll over from the fetal position onto his back so I could stretch him. I did only three stretches—the Ham-string Floor Stretch, the Piriformis Stretch and the Hip Flexors Stretch—but these were enough to loosen him up. A few minutes later he was able to get up and go to the bathroom (which had been a real problem) and then get into bed. "I definitely feel looser," Steve told me then. "My pain was a ten, and now it's down to a six or seven."

What also went down was his fear.

I came back the next day to stretch him some more, and I got him to walk down the stairs and to walk around outside, taking baby steps, one at a time. He was in shock that my simple stretches had worked so well, as he hadn't been out of bed for days. The pain wasn't gone, but it had become manageable, and he was able to do his routine tasks and go to the bathroom.

The next day Steve had an MRI and found out he had a herniated disk. His orthopedist prescribed steroids to lessen the inflammation, and in a short time Steve was able to taper off and then stop taking the potent painkillers. That night, Steve called to tell me the diagnosis and ended by saying, "When you have time, come over and teach me everything. I need to know how to live with my back!" I have to admit it was very gratifying to hear that from a physician.

It's No Joke that Coughing, Sneezing and Laughing Can Cause Back Pain

A cough, sneeze or bout of laughter can come on without warning and set your back on fire. And there's nothing funny about that!

There's not much you can do about an involuntary reaction, like a cough or a sneeze, but if you do feel one coming on and have a few seconds to get ready for it, be sure to instantly contract your abdominals and try to brace yourself against something sturdy. If you're standing, contract your abdominals and go into a slight squat. Do the same when you're in a comedy club or watching or hearing something funny. Just be conscious of your posture (don't slouch in your chair!), and try to keep your abdominals contracted as much as possible.

Stand Tall, Sit Tall, Walk Tall: How Posture Impacts Your Back Pain

There's a popular myth that as we age, we are doomed to get shorter. This happens to some people, particularly those with osteoporosis, which causes bone loss and shrinkage. But many others do not get shorter. It only appears that way thanks to poor posture.

Poor posture can be caused by many things, such as inherited conditions, injury or disease, but for most people, poor posture is a direct result of repeated bad habits. Count me in as one of the guilty ones, which is why I needed Cara to sort me out in the first place!

Few people know how to walk properly, and few always remember to keep their head up and their spine in a strong, neutral position. We slump and slouch and don't stretch. We wear heels that have us teetering forward. We tend to carry babies and bags and even backpacks on one side, which can cause our muscles to become weak and tight, eventually pulling on our poor joints so much that our structural alignment gets out of whack.

The Posture Test

❶ Stand with your back against a wall, making sure that the back of your head is touching the wall. Move your feet forward slightly so your heels are about six inches from the wall.

❷ With your buttocks touching the wall, stick your hand between your lower back and the wall, and then between your neck and the wall.

❸ If there is only an inch or two between your lower back and the wall and only two inches between your neck and the wall, your posture is good. If not, we will work on getting you to stand tall and straight!

Proper Body Alignment

Standing and Walking

❶ Stand in front of a full-length mirror. Your head should be straight, your shoulders should be back and relaxed, and your arms should be down at your sides.

❷ Your hips should be level. Place your feet directly below your hips, and balance your weight evenly.

❸ Lift your chest up and contract your abdominals.

❹ Turn sideways. You should be able to draw a straight line from your head to your toes. If so, you are properly aligned.

❺ Always try to maintain this proper alignment whenever you stand or walk.

Sitting

❶ Lead with your buttocks when you're about to sit down. Make sure your abdominals are contracted.

❷ Sit with your back in a neutral position so that all three curves (cervical, or neck; thoracic, or mid-back; and lumbar, or lower back) are aligned. This neutral spine position—with your head facing straight on, your eyes forward, your shoulders back and your buttocks touching the back of the chair—minimizes the stress on your spine. Don't slump.

❸ If you don't have an adjustable chair, place a foot rest, stool or even a thick book under your feet so they can remain flat, with your knees at a ninety-degree angle. This will keep your knees in an ideal position, aligned with your hips.

❹ Try to keep your weight evenly distributed on both legs and hips. When you feel yourself getting stiff, it's time to get up and move around, to stretch or to have a short walk. Walk around, stretch or do whatever you please. Just get up and move. If you can't get up every thirty minutes, try to move around in your seat a bit.

❺ Try contracting your abdominals every so often. This will remind you to keep your back protected and to not hunch forward.

❻ If you have to turn to get something, make sure you use your whole body to turn (that means your legs, too). Contract your abdominals, and try to brace yourself with the chair.

TIP: For more information about sitting at work, see Chapter 6.

Sleeping or Lying Down

For tips on sleeping and lying down, see Chapter 5.

Stop the Slouch

Who doesn't slouch? I'm guilty of it, and many surgeons I know are, too. It's just too easy to forget to stand tall, especially when you're tired and not aware of what you're doing until it's too late. I see this every day when people are walking down the street and texting. This is not only dangerous, but it automatically causes you to hunch over. Put the cell phone away and walk tall instead!

Slouching is one of those things that you can control (or not!). It's a terrible position as it puts you out of alignment and can unwittingly cause pain. But getting rid of the dreaded slouch takes constant reminders to sit or stand up straight.

Here's what to do:

❶ Contract your abdominals.

❷ If you're sitting in a chair, put your hands on each side and shift until your posture is realigned. Even better, stand up, think about your posture, contract your abdominals, and then sit back down and realign your body.

❸ If you're standing or walking, focus on the horizon. This will instantly elevate your head and place your spine in the neutral position, which is what proper alignment is all about.

CHAPTER 3

IMPROVING CORE STRENGTH

As you learned in Chapter 1, strengthening your entire core is an essential component of an ideal regular exercise routine for optimum back health and strength. Because all major muscle movements originate with your core, having a powerful one gives you excellent protection against back pain. It doesn't matter if you're a professional athlete, a weekend warrior, an occasional walker or someone who just likes to garden—doing a few minutes of core work several days a week is all it takes to get your muscles engaged and to make them stronger. The exercises in this chapter are an essential element of the 7-Minute Back Pain Solution and must be done along with the seven stretches.

By now, you shouldn't be surprised that there are no crunches or sit-ups in this chapter. The exercises are much better here. They work your entire core, and not just the muscles in your abdomen. All of them will help you support and protect your back.

For optimal results, you should do these exercises three or four times a week, with a day of rest in between. Always take your time with them. Quality is always more important than quantity, so always be mindful of your form and posture. The timing is really up to you. Beginners may take longer to get through the sequence. You may need to take breaks in between each exercise, especially if this is your first time doing these types of movements. Don't get discouraged if you can do only a couple of repetitions or sets. Do what you can, and then try again later in the day or the following day. Every little bit will make your core stronger.

When you have mastered these exercises and feel confident, you can increase the repetitions.

The more you do these exercises, the more acquainted you will become with the positions and how they make you feel. You know your body better than anyone, so trust yourself not to push beyond your limit—and trust this book to help guide you.

Always Concentrate on Your Form

- Be sure to follow all instructions exactly.

- Aim for a neutral spine position throughout. That means your neck, chest and lower back are in alignment. See p.74 for how to achieve the neutral spine position.

- Do not go for the burn! You should feel tension in the muscles, *not* pain. One of the worst exercise phrases ever coined is "No pain, no gain." Pushing through pain to finish an exercise or a sport is a recipe for disaster. Pain is a signal from your body that something is wrong. If any exercise causes discomfort or pain, stop doing it!

- When you breathe, inhale through your nose and exhale through your mouth. Just breathe naturally, in a way that makes you feel calm and comfortable. Never, ever hold your breath.

- Make sure you have warmed up for at least five to ten minutes before doing these exercises, to avoid any muscle strain.

- There are a few exercises that can be done on a stability ball, but if that's not possible, follow the instructions for the alternatives.

- These exercises are going to help you develop core strength, which will help your lower back pain and improve your body. Don't stress about them. And certainly don't compare yourself to anyone else.

- Again, if any exercise causes discomfort, don't do it! Be smart and sensible by going at your own pace and building up your strength without hurting your back. Every time you do these exercises, you will get a little bit stronger.

Stretches between the Exercises

Do these stretches if your back feels tense during or after the exercises.

1. Child's Pose Stretch

1 Kneel on the floor, your arms resting loosely on your thighs. Breathe normally.

2 On the exhale, contract your abdominals and slowly slide your arms forward, palms facing down, gently easing your torso forward until your head is resting on the floor.

3 Remain in the stretch for three to five seconds, then slowly rise up back to the kneeling position.

2. Cat Stretch

1 Get on your hands and knees, inhale, and then, on the exhale, contract your abdominals.

2 Slowly arch your back up toward the ceiling and lower your head. Your upper back should be higher than your shoulders.

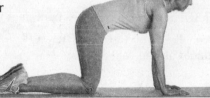

3 Hold this position for three to five seconds, and then slowly return to the starting position.

PHASE I—CORE EXERCISES

These exercises should be done daily. Use the number of repetitions and sets called for in the instructions as your guideline. Build up gradually. Always be sure to warm up for five to ten minutes and keep your abdominals contracted throughout the exercises.

Before You Start #1:
Find Your Neutral Spine Position

1 Lie with your back on the floor, knees bent, and then place your hands on top of your pelvis, just below your waist.

2 Slowly roll your pelvis forward slightly (arching your back slightly off the mat), and then slowly roll your pelvis backward gently (flattening your back on the mat).

3 Release that position. Your back should be neither arched nor completely flat on the mat to be in neutral. This should feel comfortable, not forced.

1. Abdominal Contraction

1 Lie on your back, knees bent, feet flat on the floor, and place your hands on your belly. Relax and make sure you are breathing normally. Your spine should be neutral.

2 Inhale, and then, on the exhale, contract your abdominals. Hold the contraction for ten seconds, and then release.

3 Do this five to ten times.

4 You should feel a tightening feeling around your midsection.

2. Pelvic Tilt

1 Lie on your back, knees bent, feet flat on the floor, arms at your sides, palms facedown. Relax and make sure you are breathing normally.

2 Inhale, and then, on the exhale, contract your abdominals and tilt your pelvis back. This maneuver will slightly press your back into the mat. Be sure to do it gently.

3 Hold the contraction and position for three to five seconds, and then release it slowly.

4 Do this five to ten times.

3. Abdominal Contraction with Foot Up

1 Lie on your back, knees bent, feet flat on the floor, arms at your sides, palms facedown. Relax and make sure you are breathing normally.

2 Inhale, and then, on the exhale, contract your abdominals and hold the contraction while lifting your left foot one to two inches off the floor, lower your left foot, and then lift your right foot up. Hold each foot up for two seconds.

3 Do this ten times with each foot.

4 Do two to three sets.

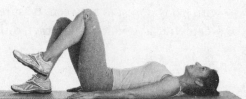

4. Abdominal Contraction with Knee Up

1 Lie on your back, knees bent, feet flat on the floor, arms at your sides, palms facedown. Relax and make sure you are breathing normally.

2 Inhale, and then, on the exhale, contract your abdominals and hold the contraction while raising your left knee up. Lower your left knee and raise your right knee up. Hold each knee up for two seconds.

3 Do this ten times with each knee.

4 Do two to three sets.

PHASE II—MORE CHALLENGING CORE EXERCISES

The following exercises are more challenging and should be done *only* after you have mastered Phase I. Do not push yourself too hard at first! It is okay to do fewer reps as you master these exercises. Once you start to feel confident and stronger, use your judgment to do another set of each exercise. This phase should be done three to four days a week, with a day of rest in between. Be sure to warm up for five to ten minutes. Keep your abdominals contracted throughout the exercises.

1. Alternating Leg Facedown

1 Lie facedown, legs straight, arms down at your sides.

2 Inhale, and then, on the exhale, contract your abdominals and hold the contraction throughout the exercise. Avoid any arching in your back or raising of your head.

3 Keep your head in line with your neck and spine.

4 Inhale, and then, on the exhale, lift your right leg two to four inches off the floor and hold for three to five seconds. Repeat with your left leg.

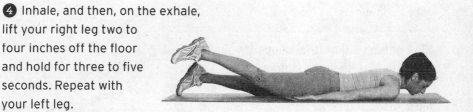

5 Do this ten times with each leg.

Optional: Child's Pose Stretch

1 Kneel on the floor, your arms resting loosely on your thighs. Breathe normally.

2 Inhale, and then, on the exhale, contract your abdominals and slowly slide your arms forward, palms facing down, gently easing your torso forward until your head is resting on the floor.

3 Remain in the stretch for three to five seconds, then slowly rise up back to the kneeling position.

2. Bridge

1 Lie on your back, knees bent, feet flat on the floor, arms at your sides, palms facedown. Relax and make sure you are breathing normally. You can place a flat pillow under your head and shoulders, if that's more comfortable. Your spine should be neutral.

2 Inhale, and then, on the exhale, contract your abdominals.

3 Tighten your buttocks and lift your hips and buttocks off the floor, pushing with your heels. Make sure your hips, knees and shoulders make a straight line.

4 Hold this position for five to eight seconds. Avoid arching your back.

5 Slowly lower yourself down.

6 Do this ten times.

3. Arm/Leg Lift on Hands and Knees

1 Start on your hands and knees, your hands should be shoulder-width apart and your knees should be hip-width apart. Inhale, and then, on the exhale, contract your abdominals and hold the contraction for five to eight seconds and release.

2 Do this five times.

3 On your hands and knees with your abdominals contracted, extend and raise your right arm off the floor and hold this position for five to eight seconds. Repeat raising your left arm.

4 Do this five times for each arm.

5 On your hands and knees with your abdominals contracted, extend and raise your right leg off the floor and hold this position for five to eight seconds. Repeat with your left leg.

6 Do this five times for each leg.

Do not let your buttocks or back rise up or your abdomen sag toward the floor. Your body should remain still throughout the exercise. Pretend that there's a full glass of water resting on your back; the water should not spill with these movements.

Keep your head level.

Optional: Cat Stretch

1 Get on your hands and knees, inhale, and then, on the exhale, contract your abdominals.

2 Slowly arch your back up toward the ceiling and lower your head. Your upper back should be higher than your shoulders.

3 Hold this position for three to five seconds, and then slowly return to the starting position.

4. Clam

❶ Lie on your left side, knees bent, your right leg atop your left leg. Place a pillow or your hand under your head for support.

❷ Contract your abdominals and then place your right arm in front of you with your hand on the floor for support.

❸ Slowly open your knees, keeping your feet together, and hold for two seconds, then slowly close your knees, while keeping your back and pelvis from moving.

❹ Repeat on your right side.

❺ Do this five to ten times with each leg.

5. Standing Alternating Arm and Knee Raise

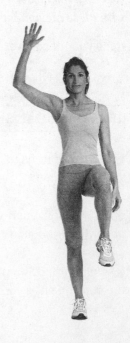

❶ Stand with your feet shoulder-width apart.

❷ Inhale, and then, on the exhale, contract your abdominals while simultaneously lifting your right arm and left knee up. Hold this position for three to five seconds, then repeat with your left arm and right knee.

❸ Do this ten times for each arm and knee.

6a. Seated Arm and Knee Raise on Stability Ball

1 Sit on a stability ball with your feet flat on the floor in front of you, hip-width apart, and your arms at your sides, or resting on the ball, if that's more comfortable.

2 Contract your abdominals as soon as you sit on the ball, and keep them contracted during the entire exercise.

3 To start, get used to sitting on the ball without rolling. This takes core strength, so make sure your abdominals are contracted.

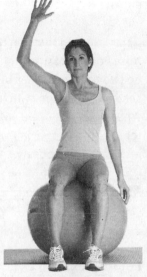

4 To find your neutral spine position, contract your abdominals, roll your pelvis slightly back and forth, and then stop in between the two positions. You should be sitting comfortably on the ball.

5 Inhale, and then, on the exhale, raise your right arm. Hold this position for three to five seconds, and then switch to your left arm.

6 Do this five to ten times.

7 Inhale, and then, on the exhale, raise your right knee up. Hold this position for three to five seconds, and then switch to your left knee.

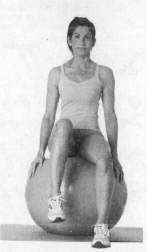

8 Do this ten times.

6b. Seated Alternating Arm and Knee Raise on Stability Ball

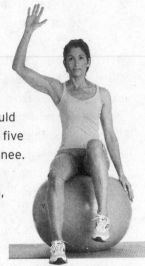

1 Sit on a stability ball with your feet flat on the floor in front of you, hip-width apart, and your arms at your sides, or resting on the ball, if that's more comfortable.

2 Contract your abdominals as soon as you sit on the ball, and keep them contracted during the entire exercise.

3 Inhale, and then, on the exhale, simultaneously raise your right arm and left knee. Your left foot should be two to three inches off the floor. Hold for three to five seconds, and then switch to your left arm and right knee. When you raise one arm, you can use the other arm for support on the ball, but if you feel steady enough, just let it hang loosely.

4 Do this ten times.

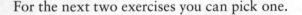

For the next two exercises you can pick one.

7. Wall Sit

1 Stand with your back flat against a wall, feet hip-width apart, and your arms at your sides.

2 Walk your feet about two feet away from the wall.

3 Keep your back flat against the wall, and contract your abdominals. Then slowly squat down until your knees are at a forty-five-degree angle, putting yourself into a comfortable squat. You should load the weight on your heels as you come down. Hold this position for five to ten seconds.

4 Place your hands on the wall for support and slowly push yourself up.

5 Do this five to ten times.

To advance this exercise you can squat to a ninety-degree angle, while doing this exercise.

8. Wall Squat with Stability Ball

1 Place the stability ball against a wall and gently lean against it, feet hip-width apart, hands on your waist. The ball should rest against the small of your back, with your mid-back and lower back making contact with the ball.

2 Walk your feet about six to twelve inches away from the wall.

3 Inhale, and then, on the exhale, contract your abdominals and slowly squat down. You will be leaning into the ball as you come down, loading the weight on your heels. Hold this position for five to ten seconds.

4 Inhale, and then, on the exhale, slowly push back up to the starting position.

5 Do this ten times.

PHASE III—THE MOST CHALLENGING CORE EXERCISES

The following exercises are even more challenging and should be done *only* after you have mastered Phase I and Phase II. Start with the modified versions of the exercises, and gradually build up your strength before progressing to the more difficult exercises. Do not push yourself too hard at first! It is okay to do fewer reps as you master these exercises. This phase should be done three to four times a week, with a day of rest in between. Once you start to feel confident and stronger, use your judgment to do another set of each exercise. Be sure to warm up for five to ten minutes. Keep your abdominals contracted throughout the exercises.

1. Alternating Arm and Opposite Straight Leg, Facedown

❶ Lie facedown with your legs straight and your arms extended flat on the floor in front of you.

❷ Inhale, and then, on the exhale, contract your abdominals and hold the contraction throughout the exercise. Avoid any arching in your back or raising of your head.

❸ Inhale, and then, on the exhale, lift your right arm and left leg two to four inches off the floor.

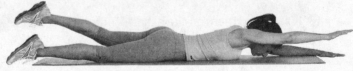

❹ Hold this position for three to five seconds. Switch to your left arm and right leg and repeat.

❺ Do this ten times.

Optional: Child's Pose Stretch

1 Kneel on the floor, your arms resting loosely on your thighs. Breathe normally.

2 Inhale, and then, on the exhale, contract your abdominals and slowly slide your arms forward, palms facing down, gently easing your torso forward until your head is resting on the floor.

3 Remain in the stretch for three to five seconds, then slowly rise up back to the kneeling position.

2. Plank on Knees

1 Lie on the floor facedown, resting on your elbows and knees.

2 Inhale, and then, on the exhale, contract your abdominals and tighten your buttocks.

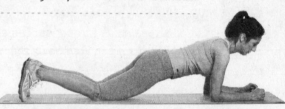

3 Lift your feet up off the floor so that you are still resting on your elbows and knees.

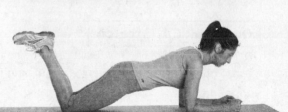

4 Hold this position for five to eight seconds. Keep your shoulders, hips and knees in a straight line.

5 Do this ten times.

3. Alternating Arm with Opposite Leg on Hands and Knees

1 Start on your hands and knees. Inhale, and then, on the exhale, contract your abdominals.

2 Lift your right arm and left leg simultaneously.

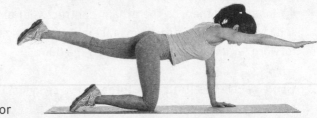

3 Hold the extension for five to eight seconds, and then lower your right arm and left leg. Switch to your left arm and right leg and repeat.

4 Do this ten times.

Do not let your buttocks or back rise or your abdomen sag toward the floor. Your body should remain still throughout the exercise. Pretend that there's a full glass of water resting on your back; the water should not spill with these movements.

Optional: Cat Stretch

1 Get on your hands and knees, inhale, and then, on the exhale, contract your abdominals.

2 Slowly arch your back up toward the ceiling and lower your head. Your upper back should be higher than your shoulders.

3 Hold this position for three to five seconds, and then slowly return to the starting position.

4. Side Plank on Knees

1 Lie on your right side, propped up by your right elbow. Bend both knees at a ninety-degree angle, with your left foot resting atop your right foot.

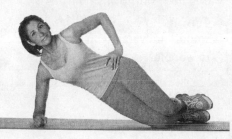

2 Contract your abdominals, and slowly raise your body up to support your weight on your right arm. Your right elbow should bend at ninety degrees directly under your shoulder. Place your left hand on your waist. If you need more support, place your left hand on the floor in front of you.

3 Tighten your buttocks and slowly lift your hips up off the floor. Hold this position for five to eight seconds, then slowly lower your hips.

4 Do this ten times on each side.

5. Hamstring on Stability Ball

1 Lie on your back, placing the backs of your lower legs and heels on top of a stability ball. Your legs will be straight. Your feet should be hip-width apart on top of the ball with your toes pointed toward the ceiling.

2 Inhale, and then, on the exhale, contract your abdominals and tighten your buttocks. Slowly lift up until your hips, legs and torso form a straight line. Your lower back should be

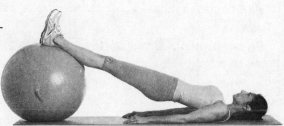

lifted a few inches off the floor, while your shoulders and upper back stay on the floor. Avoid lifting your body too high when bridging, and don't drop too low when bringing the ball toward you. If you feel any pressure on your shins, readjust your feet.

3 With your abdominals contracted, slowly pull your knees in toward your chest (rolling the ball toward you), and then slowly push the ball away with your toes. This is a smooth movement so try not to wobble.

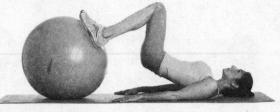

4 Do this ten to fifteen times.

6. Alternating Arm with Opposite Leg on Stability Ball

1 Lie on your stomach over the ball. Your hands and feet should be on the floor.

2 Inhale, and then, on the exhale, contract your abdominals while simultaneously lifting up your right arm and left knee. Hold this position for four to six seconds, then repeat with your left arm and right knee.

3 Do this ten times.

Be careful not to arch your back.

The next two exercises are more advanced. Do them *only* if you are able to master the previous Plank exercises.

7. Plank

1 Lie on the floor facedown, resting on your elbows and knees.

2 Inhale, and then, on the exhale, contract your abdominals and tighten your buttocks.

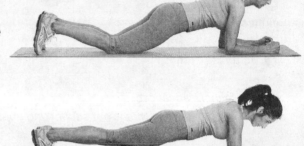

3 Slowly rise up and shift your weight back on your toes. You should be balancing on your elbows and toes. Your elbows should be aligned with your shoulders. Avoid any arching of your lower back. Make sure your buttocks don't rise up—your body should be in a straight line with your abdominal muscles contracted throughout the exercise.

4 Hold this position for eight seconds, and then slowly lower yourself.

5 Do this five to ten times.

8. Side Plank

1 Lie on your right side, propped up by your right elbow, legs straight, your left foot resting either atop your right foot or slightly in front of it for support. Place your left hand on your waist or on the mat in front of you, if you need the extra support.

2 Inhale, and then, on the exhale, contract your abdominals and tighten your buttocks.

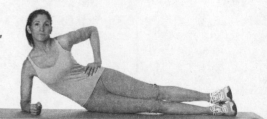

3 Raise your hips and knees up using your core and your right arm. Your right elbow should be bent at a ninety-degree angle.

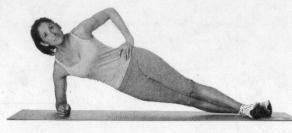

4 Hold this position for eight seconds.

5 Do this ten times.

If you are more advanced,
you can lift up the arm that is not supporting you.

Follow all of these exercises with the seven stretches.

PART

2

The 7-Minute Back Pain Solution and Your Daily Life

CHAPTER 4

MANAGING YOUR BACK PAIN AT HOME

THIS CHAPTER COVERS THE BASICS about how to move with back pain when you're dealing with the necessary, often daily chores you need to do around the house. What's most important to remember with these chores—which often seem benign, because you're so used to doing them (and so tired of doing them, too!)—is that they can be a real pain in the neck. And back!

Boring, tedious and never-ending tasks can be the ones to set your back off, because most people are rarely conscious of how they're using their bodies when they dust the bookshelves, push a vacuum around the living room, get the clothes out of the dryer or plant some tomatoes in the garden. These are repetitive motions that involve pushing, pulling, lifting, carrying, bending, twisting and/or reaching. Worse, they're often done continuously over a period of time, but because you're most likely thinking about getting the chores done as quickly as possible, instead of thinking about your back, you can unwittingly put yourself at risk for more pain.

Because the mechanics behind how to do chores properly isn't a "sexy" topic, it is rarely discussed. But it should be. Household chores and cleaning are tasks that demand attention and never end (and sometimes seem endless), but our philosophy is that your back is more important than dusting. To be sure, no one wants to live in a dirty house, but you want to protect your back in order to prevent any injuries that might not let you clean again for a period of time (just think of all the dusting *then!*). In other words, a very small amount of pre-cleaning preparation, as well as a consciousness of how you are moving, go an extremely long way in making your chores more manageable as well as pain free.

In Chapter 3, you found the core exercises that will strengthen the muscles you use most in everyday life. Doing these exercises will not bulk you up like a weight lifter in a gym. Instead, the purpose of this training is to make your tasks easier and quicker, with less strain on your back. Strengthening your entire body always helps take the stress off your back.

We want to teach you a new language of simple movements that minimize stress on your back and help you get your everyday tasks done with maximum efficiency, so we've broken all these tasks down into easy steps. Follow them exactly. They might look detailed at first, but they are all very simple. After doing them just a few times, they should become second nature to you.

Cleaning Basics That Will Help to Protect Your Back

❶ Plan ahead. Make a schedule and keep the information handy. Always make a note when you need to replenish cleaning supplies.

❷ Try not to clean the whole house at once. For example, you can clean the downstairs one day and the upstairs the next. If you have only one day to do it, though, break up the chores. Clean several rooms, then take a break and do something that keeps you moving but isn't stressful for your back (go out and walk the dog, for example), and then stretch. Do your vacuuming last, as it will be less stressful if your body is already warmed up from the other cleaning.

❸ Avoid spending a lot of time on only one chore, especially one with a repetitive motion, like sweeping or vacuuming. Break it up as much as possible. Try dusting for ten to fifteen minutes, take a break, and then either go back to dusting or move on to mopping and vacuuming.

④ Remember to keep your feet shoulder-width apart when doing any chores that require standing, like dusting. Be conscious of your posture.

⑤ If you have to lift anything, keep your knees bent. Use the power of your legs, not your back. Don't lift heavy objects by yourself!

⑥ Avoid twisting.

⑦ Contract your abdominals as much as you can, and breathe normally.

⑧ Wear comfortable clothes and footwear.

⑨ Take your time! Rushing through chores means you aren't concentrating on your back. Slow and steady will save you plenty of time later as you won't have to nurse your back.

⑩ Stretch when you are done cleaning.

⑪ Remember that no matter how much you clean today, you'll still have cleaning to do in the future. It is much better to have a strong, pain-free back than a shiny floor!

How to Choose Tools That Are the Least Stressful for Your Back

Look for tools with large or wide handles for kitchen, bathroom and outdoor chores. These will be less stressful for your back due to physics (area and pressure are inversely related). If a tool has a small handle, the pressure (and force) transmitted increases, which in turn increases the forces on your body. If, on the other hand, a tool has a handle—like that on a toothbrush or a can opener—loading and pinch grip forces are reduced.

Whenever possible, look for handles that can be attached, as they eliminate the need to bend over and help your posture, and you know by now that bending over to do chores or to pull something automatically puts your back in a less than optimum position. Whoever invented rolling luggage with extendable handles has saved countless people from low back pain! And whoever invented handles or extenders that can be attached to different tools also deserves a medal.

If you are interested in finding more back-friendly and ergonomically designed tools for use around the house and garden, do a search for "assistive devices," "assistive technology" and "activities of daily living." You'll find a wide variety of websites with useful information and products.

IN THE HOUSE

Housework

When your back hurts, cleaning is probably the last thing you want to do . . . but if your house gets messy, that can cause stress, which can in turn trigger back pain. Follow these tips, and you can keep up with the chores without putting your back at risk.

❶ When you aren't in pain, organize your heavy and most used cleaning supplies so they are easy to reach. A great idea is to use a lightweight plastic caddy or a bucket for supplies. Don't overload it, but add as many items as you can lift without straining. Keeping all the supplies in one container will minimize bending under the sink or twisting to reach shelves to get them.

❷ When you have back pain, realize that you might not get everything done, so do what's most important first. Dusting and window washing can wait!

❸ Always bend with your knees bent (squat position). Avoid bending or twisting at the waist when your legs are straight. Always contract your abdominals when lifting, pushing, pulling or carrying.

❹ When reaching for things in cupboards, keep your abdominals contracted and lift your heels off the floor and go up on your toes. Don't strain to reach anything. Keep a sturdy stepladder handy, and use it to minimize the risk of back strain.

❺ Take back breaks when you can. Don't underestimate how physical this kind of work can be. Do the seven-minute stretches, and try to walk around to help loosen up the muscles further; or reverse it, and walk around for a few minutes before stretching.

❻ Change your positions while doing chores at the sink or stove so you don't get stiff and possibly hurt your back. A footstool is a handy tool as you can rest a foot on it while you're standing. We'll show you how to use your arms, legs and core muscles when doing chores to take the strain off your back.

❼ Remember to breathe properly. Housework is still exertion, and sometimes we hold our breath without realizing it.

How to Incorporate Housework into Your Strength and Core Regimen

It's a lot easier to tackle annoying chores when you look at the time spent as a substitute for the time you'd spend doing strengthening, body-toning exercises! These steps might seem a bit time-consuming at first, but trust us, they aren't. You'll quickly master them, saving your back from hurting, and getting your chores done more efficiently.

Vacuuming

This task can cause a lot of back pain because you are usually hunched over, and you're doing a repetitive motion with a vibrating piece of equipment that can be heavy. Lugging the vacuum around can be hard on your back if done improperly. Look for lightweight vacuums with long cords, or plug the vacuum into an extension cord. The less you have to stoop down to deal with the plug, the better.

❶ Stand upright, contract your abdominals, and use your arms and legs—not your back!—when pushing and pulling a vacuum cleaner.

❷ Use a lunge position when vacuuming, relying on the vacuum for support. Place one foot in front, shift your weight onto that foot, and then push off with your back foot. Use this position as you go back and forth.

❸ Vacuum one side of the carpet or rug; then turn and come back in the other direction. This might take a bit longer, but it avoids the push/pull motion, which can affect your lower back.

❹ Stairs can be tricky, so take your time and hold on to the railing with one hand. It is not advisable to use a heavy vacuum or an upright vacuum on stairs. It's much better to use a canister-type vacuum with the attachment hose. Bend your knees slightly, and then go up the steps, keeping one foot on one step and the other on the step below it. Be sure not to hunch over.

❺ If you don't have a problem with your knees, you can try kneeling on each step (you might want to use a knee pad) when vacuuming stairs. Make sure your abdominals are contracted. Do not, however, do this with an upright vacuum. Only the canister type with an attachment hose is suitable.

❻ You can also sit on each step as you go, vacuuming the step below you.

Mopping and Sweeping

Mopping and sweeping are also tough on your back, as you tend to hunch over while in motion. Often, you don't realize how much back strain you've caused until you are done with your chores and stand up straight to put the tools away.

Mopping

❶ Look for a mop with a long handle. If possible, use the sink to wring it out and rewet it. Using a bucket on the floor means bending over to get to it. If you must use a bucket, be sure to squat down, instead of bending.

❷ When using a mop, make sure your abdominals are contracted and you are standing upright. Keep your knees slightly bent. And keep the mop close to you when working with it. Don't reach too far forward with it.

❸ Try to keep moving when mopping so you're not tempted to overstretch with the mop. You can always go back over spots you missed. Do small sections at a time.

❹ You can move the mop from side to side or in little circles. Just make sure your abdominals are contracted and your knees are slightly bent. Keep breathing!

❺ This might sound a little nutty at first, but it really works—and it gives your legs a great workout. Try cleaning the floor with your feet instead, as it's a great lower body workout. You can do this either with an old pair of sneakers or bare feet, and with towels or cloths saturated with cleanser or with the cleanser poured directly on the floor. (If you're worried about harsh chemicals touching your feet, this is a good time to switch to eco-friendly products, or use the cheapest and safest cleaner around: white vinegar diluted with water.) Place damp small to medium towels under your feet, contract your abdominals, keeping your knees slightly bent, and then get moving, as if you are ice-skating or rollerblading. As you move about, you can lean on the countertops for support, if you feel you need to; just be sure not to hunch over. When you clean this way, you really feel it in your legs! Don't overdo it at first. Do small areas until you're confident with the motion. And when you're done, be sure to take off your wet sneakers or dry your feet so you don't slip or get anything wet.

Sweeping

❶ When sweeping, stand upright and keep your abdominals contracted.

❷ If you need to twist to the side, bend your knees and use your arms and legs to do so.

❸ If you need to get down to floor level to use a dustpan, do so by bending your knees and gently squatting.

❹ Overreaching causes stress on the back, so avoid it when you can. Try not to bend at the waist with your legs straight; always keep your knees bent slightly.

❺ Try to switch your hand placement on the broom (or mop) from time to time.

Dusting

One thing about dusting—as soon as you do it, doesn't it seem as if the dust instantly comes back? Even this seemingly benign activity can have serious repercussions for your back if you do it too quickly or improperly.

1 With the dusting cloth in your hand, contract your abdominals and breathe. Don't bend at the waist with your legs straight; always keep your knees slightly bent.

2 If you are dusting a piece of furniture at chest level, try to lean against it when reaching to dust. Switch hands whenever possible.

3 If a piece of furniture is low, squat down and place one hand on your thigh or the furniture for support if you need to.

4 Try not to reach too far. Get as close as possible to whatever it is you're dusting.

5 When your back is really hurting, realize that the dusting is not a vital chore (unless you have asthma). Don't push it!

6 When reaching up to dust something, lift your heels off the floor and go up on your toes, rather than overstretching your arms. Use a step stool, if possible.

Doing the Laundry

1 Plan ahead. Arrange heavy detergent bottles so they are easy to get to. Avoid having to reach for them, but if you do, use your feet. Lift your heels and go up on your toes.

2 Never overload your laundry bag or basket. Try using a backpack that has long, wide straps and that sits high on your back, or use a rolling duffel bag. If you prefer a basket, carry it close to your body at chest level, and keep your abdominals contracted while carrying it.

3 If possible, place the basket or laundry bag on the dryer or on a table when sorting your clothes, as you want to avoid bending over. Keep it within easy reach. If that's not possible, squat down when transferring clothes to the machines. If you prefer to stand, you can place your hand on top of the machines for support, or use a footstool when putting clothes in or taking them out. If you do have to lift the basket up from the floor, make sure you contract your abdominals, squat down, bring the basket to chest height and then slowly rise.

4 Wet clothes are heavier, so when unloading your washing machine, take only a few pieces out at a time. Always keep your abdominals contracted and knees bent, rather than bending over with your legs straight. You can also lean your hand on the machine for support or use a footstool.

5 If you have a front-loading washer or dryer, make sure to squat rather than bend over when placing clothes in the machine. If you have a top-loading machine, bend your knees when loading clothes into it.

6 Try not to twist your body with your basket or bag in hand, but if you have to, pivot your foot first and then turn your body.

IN THE BATHROOM
At the Sink: Brushing Your Teeth and Washing Your Face

When you're in pain, even the smallest daily movements can trouble your back—and it's the ones you don't even think about that can make things worse, as you don't even know what you've done to exacerbate the pain. One thing we've noticed is that people tend to hunch over when at the sink. They also tend to bend over or twist with their legs straight. You always want to avoid doing that. Keep your knees slightly bent.

1 Contract your abdominals, and bend your knees slightly. Avoid bending over at the waist with your legs straight.

2 Try not to twist too much with any of your motions.

❸ If you are very short, you might want to use a small stool so you can look in the mirror without straining. If you're tall, remember not to hunch.

❹ For extra support at the sink, stack hand towels on both sides of the basin so that you can rest your arms while leaning very slightly over, keeping your knees slightly bent, to brush your teeth and wash your face. Make sure the towels are the right height for your arms so you're not uncomfortable. You can also stack the towels in front of your pelvic area to prevent you from leaning over the basin too much. Sinks are often too low for your height, causing you to lean forward over them, which you don't want to do.

❺ When brushing your teeth, you don't have to stand at the sink. Since we're supposed to brush for two minutes, anyway, try walking around so you're not in the same position for a long time. Cara likes to walk around the house, shutting off the lights, checking on the dog, and putting the alarm on, while brushing at night. In the morning she brushes while going downstairs to get the coffee going. It's good for your back and your teeth!

On the Toilet

This is a tough topic for many people to talk about, but you should not feel embarrassed when dealing with the fact that getting on and off the toilet multiple times each day can be something you dread when you're in pain.

The biggest problem with toilets is that you have to sit on them. And what does sitting do for so many back-pain sufferers? It causes more pain. So remember, sitting on the toilet is still sitting. Worse, a toilet tends to be low to the floor. Plus, there's a hole in the middle, so you have no back support whatsoever. This is a posture buster before you've even lowered your derriere! Follow these tips, and you won't have to worry anymore.

TIP: The most important thing to remember is to use your arms and legs as much as possible to support your weight, so you're not using your back.

TIP: Women have an advantage, as it is much easier to manage a skirt than deal with pulling pants up and down when you have back pain. If you are home and can wear casual clothing, try to wear outfits that have as few fastenings as possible and that are super easy to put on and take off. This way you'll avoid excess motion and twisting.

TIP: Keeping your feet elevated while you are on the toilet will instantly relieve some of the stress on your back, because by elevating your feet, you align your knees with your hips. A child's stool works well for this because it is nonslip.

TIP: Installing handles in the bathroom will provide extra support that will help you to get up and down more easily.

How to Sit Down on the Toilet

❶ Make sure the toilet paper is easily accessible and that you do not have to twist your body around or reach to get it. (In most homes and public restrooms, it is not!) You may want to invest in a toilet paper caddy, as this will minimize reaching.

❷ Stand as close to the toilet as possible and contract your abdominals.

❸ Slowly squat down, lean forward slightly and stick your buttocks out a bit. As soon as your hands can reach it, grasp the sides of the toilet seat. You will instantly feel better, as this action takes the weight off your back and enables you to better brace yourself.

❹ Slowly ease yourself down, keeping your hands on the toilet seat if you still need the extra support.

❺ If you have a stool, use it to prop up your feet. If you're in a public restroom, you might find it more comfortable to point your toes down, which will elevate your heel. You can even slip your feet out of your shoes and rest your feet on your shoes or your handbag. (The point is that even a very slight amount of elevation helps take pressure off your back.)

6 To avoid sitting down, try squatting over the toilet bowl, with your hands on your thighs, or with one hand on one thigh and the other hand braced against the wall. Only do this if this position doesn't make you feel uncomfortable and you feel that your weight is supported. It's actually a great technique, as it takes the pressure off your back and removes the worry that you'll have trouble getting up and down.

Getting Up from the Toilet

1 If you're wearing pants, pull them up as high as possible before you stand up, as the less you have to tug or bend over, the better.

2 Use your hands to help push you up, with knees bent, place your hands palms down on your thighs. Walk your hands up your legs as you stand. Or you can place your hands in between your legs on the toilet seat and then use them to help push you up. Place one hand at a time on your legs as you slowly straighten up. Your pants should already be up to thigh level, so you shouldn't have to bend over to finish pulling them up.

3 If you have a cane, don't be shy about using it to give you additional support when getting up. It can make a huge difference to have something to brace your weight right next to the toilet.

TIP: If you are out and need to use a public restroom, choose a handicapped stall, as these are outfitted with additional railings to help you brace yourself when getting up and down.

Don't Be Squeamish—Constipation and Back Pain Is a Touchy Topic, but Let's Talk About Why You Need to Deal with It

No one really likes to talk about the elimination factor, but if you are constipated, you're already feeling crummy. What makes matters worse is that some of the medications that many people take for back pain increase constipation. In addition, those who are constipated often need to spend long periods on the toilet, in what is an uncomfortable and unnatural sitting position. Straining while on the toilet increases the pressure on your lower back muscles and can cause them to tense up—which, as you know by now, can mean more lower back pain.

We spoke to Fairfield, Connecticut, gastroenterologist Dr. Julie Spivack about the relationship between your bowels and back pain, and she had these comments:

"While a brief time on the toilet is unlikely to cause major back strain, sitting on one for an extended period can be bad for your back, especially if straining to move bowels is involved. You do need abdominal muscles to help push out stool. If the muscles are weak, stool will need to be very soft so that it passes easily without requiring increased intra-abdominal pressure.

"With constipation, however, you increase intra-abdominal pressure when you strain, and that results in more pressure on your lower spine. A potent link between back pain and GI problems is the constipation that develops if someone is taking narcotics to alleviate their back pain. Narcotic-induced constipation (also called narcotic bowel) can be very severe, and often people will sit and strain for long periods of time, which is bad for lower back muscles and results in a vicious cycle.

"The best position for elimination is to allow gravity to be working with you. You also need to be able to relax your pelvic floor muscles to straighten the rectum and allow for elimination. Thus the normal position on a toilet bowl isn't bad for elimination, but sitting at ninety degrees or slouching puts strain on your lower back, so you don't want to sit at this angle for an extended period of time. Squatting is probably better, but it's difficult for people to do.

"Basically, the worst thing you can do, especially if you have lower back pain, is to ignore the urge to move your bowels because the timing or location is 'inconvenient.' This can lead to withholding stool and an inability to relax your pelvic floor muscles when you are ready to sit on the toilet.

"The best thing you can do to improve this situation, especially if you have lower back pain and constipation, is to increase the fiber in your diet, increase fluid intake, increase overall activity/exercise, don't delay in going to the bathroom when you have the urge, strengthen the pelvic floor muscles, with Kegel exercises, take a daily probiotic, which can alleviate bloating and constipation in some people, and don't obsess over your bowels, as there is no reason to force yourself to move them every day. And, of course, strengthen your abdominal muscles and back muscles."

Getting In and Out of Bathtubs and Showers

Bathtubs

Many people enjoy a long therapeutic soak in hot water when their back or muscles are aching. But bathtubs and back pain can be a tricky proposition, so I don't recommend that you take baths when your back pain is acute, as getting in and out of the tub can be difficult. And bathtubs are always slippery and wet after use, and a fall can be catastrophic, even if you don't have back pain. Never get in a tub that does not have a large nonslip mat or decals on the bottom, and make sure all your essentials (towel, robe, soap and shampoo) are within reach before you turn the water on.

❶ A cane or a stick can help tremendously with balance. You can use it to help brace your weight as you get in and out of the tub. Be sure to place it next to the tub before you start!

❷ Be careful when leaning down to turn on the faucets. Fold a towel, slowly place it on the floor, and then slowly lower yourself so you are on your knees. Inch closer to the faucets, turn them on, and then slowly get up off your knees. Use the side of the tub to brace your arms. Or try sitting as close to the faucets as possible on the edge of the tub. That way, you won't have to twist, as you'll be sitting sideways already.

❸ When getting in the tub, you want to avoid any more twisting of your torso than is necessary. To do this, very slowly step in sideways.

④ As soon as your hands can grip the sides of the tub, use this support to lower yourself all the way down. Contract your abdominals, bend your knees slightly, and then lower yourself into a seated position in the tub.

⑤ When getting out of the tub, slowly get on all fours, if this doesn't bother your knees, contract your abdominals, place your hands on the sides of the tub for support so that when you lift yourself up it's easier, and then shift your weight first to one leg and then to the other to come up straight.

⑥ Make sure there is a nonskid bath mat or rug next to the tub for you to step onto after your bath.

Showers

The hot water of a shower can feel good on your back, and it can also warm up your muscles. But getting into the shower stall or tub involves some amount of twisting and stepping.

① Be sure that your shampoo and soap and all other supplies are in place and easily accessible before you get in. Keep a nonslip mat in the shower at all times. Have your towels as close to the shower as possible to minimize movement when you are wet.

② If you have to go over a step to get into the shower stall, move as slowly as possible. Contract your abdominals right before you take the step. Keep your knees slightly bent.

③ When turning around in the shower, use Protection Mode and pivot with your feet.

④ Don't bend over to pick anything up. Squat down, if you can. When shaving your legs, try to sit or use a footstool. This activity puts you in an awkward position, even if your back isn't hurting, so plan ahead before bending over!

IN THE KITCHEN

Some people have help with the household cleaning chores, but all my patients spend time in the kitchen, cooking, cleaning up and putting food and heavy items away. Advance planning will help your back tremendously. Always try to plan ahead *when you're not in pain* so you can think clearly, get organized and keep essentials and often-used items handy in the kitchen.

TIP: A sturdy chair with a padded cushion or a footstool goes a long way to help you in the kitchen.

Unloading the Groceries

So your bags full of food have been carefully lifted out of the car and brought into the kitchen. Now what? You already know that unpacking involves a lot of twisting as you reach into the bag, pull items out, then place them on shelves or in bins of varying heights. Not only that, but if you're like most, you want to get this chore over with, so you might not pay attention to your back until it really starts to hurt.

1 Make sure you always place your grocery bags on the counters or a table. You don't want to do any lifting from the floor if you can help it.

2 Contract your abdominals and keep breathing normally whenever you lift an item out of the bag. Use both hands, as using only one hand causes back strain, especially if the object is heavy.

3 If your back is hurting, bring a sturdy chair close to wherever your bags are, and place one knee only on the chair to brace yourself.

4 When putting an item away on a high shelf, do not reach up with your knees locked and your arms outstretched. Instead, go up on tiptoes, as this will immediately take some strain off your back. Use both hands.

Basic Cooking

Cooking can involve a surprisingly large amount of twisting and bending over. Even those with strong, pain-free backs can get a jolt when they lean down to pull a heavy roast turkey out of the oven. Be prepared, and remain conscious of how you're bending.

TIP: If you like to spend a lot of time cooking, you can take some of the strain off your feet and back by purchasing a large gel or foam chef's mat to stand on.

---

❶ If you can, plan ahead. Get all your cookware and utensils out and on the counters near you to minimize movement.

❷ When standing, always make sure your feet are shoulder-width apart. If you have to stand in the same position at the stove for an extended period of time, you might want to get a chair with a padded cushion, or fold up a towel and place it on the seat. Prop one knee up on the chair. Switch knees every few minutes. Or place your foot on the chair, as long as it isn't too high. What you want to do is avoid staying in one position for an extended period of time.

❸ Always contract your abdominals and go into a squat, with your feet shoulder-width apart and your knees slightly bent, when doing any lifting or bending. Bring the item up to your waist, keeping it as close to your body as possible, especially when you're dealing with items in an oven. (This is one of the reasons Cara loves her slow cooker. It makes cooking dinner a breeze, and as it stays on the counter, so there's no bending down and lifting.)

Washing the Dishes in the Sink, and Loading and Unloading the Dishwasher

Washing the dishes can be a real pain in the back, as you tend to be in an awkward position for a period of time, especially when you load and unload the dishwasher. Most people don't think about doing the dishes as anything other than an annoying task after dinner, but going up and down with the dishes, especially if you're bending at the waist with your legs straight, is not good for your back.

❶ If you're washing dishes at the sink, gently pull a sturdy chair as close to the sink as possible. Place one bent knee on the chair, and alternate knees every few minutes.

❷ If you're not using a chair, stand with your feet shoulder-width apart and make sure your abdominals are contracted. Try to brace yourself against the lower cabinets so you don't lean over the sink to wash the dishes. Keep your knees slightly bent.

❸ When placing dishes into the sink to be washed, chose the nearest area so you don't have to reach. You might want to invest in an over-the-sink dish rack to give you height so you don't have to reach down into the sink as much.

❹ When dealing with the dishwasher, a chair is quite useful. Place all the dirty items on the counter above the dishwasher or in your over-the-sink dish rack. Either load the dishwasher while sitting on the chair, or load it while kneeling with one leg on the chair. The leg closest to the dishwasher should remain on the floor. Reverse sides when you can.

❺ If you don't want to use a chair when loading the dishwasher, then make sure you squat down, with your abdominals contracted and your feet shoulder-width apart. Do not bend from the waist.

❻ Sit or kneel when unloading the dishwasher, too. Place all the items on the counter first before putting them away. If you don't want to use a chair, unload from the same squatting position as in step 5. Always pivot your foot first, and then turn your body to lift the dishes out of the dishwasher.

IN THE BEDROOM

Making the Bed

❶ Place one knee on top of the bed for support, contract your abdominals, and use your arms, not your back, to adjust the sheets and blanket on one side of the bed. Then switch to the other knee to do the other side of the bed.

❷ Follow the same rules when removing bedding.

❸ You can also sit on the edge of the bed, contract your abdominals, slowly turn to one side, and then lean over and either put on or take off the bedding.

④ Try not to hunch over when making or stripping the bed.

Getting Dressed

The objective here is to avoid bending over, reaching and twisting as much as possible. If you're a parent, take a tip from those toddler or school-age days, when you laid out your child's clothes the night before. If you do this for yourself, when you have time to think about what you're doing and are not in the usual morning rush, you'll be able to minimize the number of drawer openings and searches for the missing shoe at the bottom of the closet, and you'll spend less time wondering what to wear.

> **TIP:** Try to keep the clothes you wear the most in drawers or on shelves at chest height. This will help minimize the number of times you lean over every morning.

Putting on Your Socks and Shoes

These simple movements you've done tens of thousands of times before, but I'll bet you rarely think about them unless your back is throbbing. These tasks can put a tremendous amount of strain on your back.

❶ Try to sit in a sturdy chair or bed when you put on your socks and shoes. Have your shoes right next to you—*not* on the floor!

❷ Try to use a long shoehorn with a handle. This will avoid the leaning-over position, which causes back strain.

❸ Bring your leg up onto the chair or whatever you are sitting on to put your socks and shoes on. When tying your shoes, *never* bend over.

For information about How to Try on Shoes while shopping, see p. 192 in Chapter 8.

IN THE LIVING ROOM

Watching TV and Movies

Do you pay attention to how you're sitting when you're watching your favorite show or a movie at home, especially if you're deeply engrossed in what's on the screen? Chances are pretty high you're slouching or slumped over. This can wreak havoc on your back, as the longer you sit in front of a television screen without moving, the more you will feel it as soon as you get up. Even if your living room sofa or special chair is firm and comfortable, you need to shift and get up and move around whenever possible. Use the commercial breaks to move around or change your position. Or make a bet with yourself that you'll check on your sitting position every time there's a boring line of dialogue in a movie, or do some stretching during the commercials. Chances are you'll be moving and stretching a lot more often than usual!

TIP: When you buy living room furniture, remember that really soft sofas and chairs might feel comfortable at first, but excess padding for your derriere means the strain will get shifted to your back. Also check the height of sofas and chairs. When you are sitting, your knees should be in line with your hips. If a sofa or chair is too low, you will soon feel it.

TIP: Recliners can feel great, but if you put the leg rest up, don't extend your legs straight out. Always keep your knees slightly bent to avoid excess strain on your back.

IN THE DINING ROOM

At the Dining Room Table

Setting the Table

❶ As you did at the sink when washing dishes, you might want to use a chair to prop up one knee when setting the table.

❷ It's better to make more trips to and from the table than to carry too many things at once. Don't lean over the table to arrange the plates and cutlery. Walk around it instead.

❸ Load up your dishes and stemware for your table on a serving cart on wheels, so you're not running back and forth from the cabinets to the table.

Sitting at the Table

❶ If you drop something (like your napkin), think about what you need to do before reaching down for it. Move your chair out slightly, then spread your legs so that you can place one hand in the middle of the chair, and then slowly reach down. Or get up and squat down, rather than bending over at the waist.

❷ When sitting, use good posture. Make sure you are not slumping or hunching over in your chair. Sit with your shoulders back and your buttocks firmly against the back of the seat. Try keeping a footstool handy to raise your feet if you're going to be sitting for a while, or at least try to reposition yourself in your seat if you can't get up. Go ahead and fidget, contracting your abdominals and then shifting your pelvis backward and forward until you find your ideal neutral spine position.

❸ Try not to reach for items. Ask someone to pass the plate.

❹ Remember, even if you're having an enjoyable dinner, you're still sitting!

IN THE GARAGE

Lots of people like to spend many contented hours working on projects in the garage. Follow the steps outlined in the Basic Cooking section on p. 108 to avoid strain on your back. A bucket, toolbox or caddy on the workbench will help keep your tools and supplies in one place.

TIP: Do not carry your tools around your waist, if you can avoid it. Tool belts pull on your pelvis, which can put a lot of unwanted strain on your lower back muscles. Use a caddy or toolbox instead. Make sure it is not too heavy and it is easy to move around.

TIP: I am not a fan of weight-lifting belts, which a lot of people like to put on when doing heavy chores or serious weight training at the gym. These belts give you a false sense of security and can actually cause more harm than good. The reason is that this kind of belt is like an old-fashioned girdle. It does the work for you, but if your own abdominal muscles do not have to contribute, they will not get stronger. And as you know by now, that's one of the worst things for your back. Rather than wear a belt, follow our tips for proper lifting, be Back Mindful when you lift and learn how to engage your core.

IN THE YARD

Like housework you do inside the home, outdoor work can be annoying, as it's always going to be there, no matter how much you attend to it. The lawn needs mowing, the leaves need raking, the weeds need yanking and let's not get started on the havoc snow can wreak on your driveway and your back! Don't overdo it, as being a weekend garden warrior can be as dangerous for your back as being a weekend golf or jogging warrior. Be conscious of all your movements.

TIP: The weather is the first thing you should think about before going outdoors to do chores. You need to be dressed appropriately for your tasks, especially when it is cold out. After all, what's the first thing you do when you get cold? You hunch over to conserve your energy. You tense up. This is the opposite of having the nice, warm, safely stretched muscles that are the heart of this book.

Shoveling Snow

The thought of having to shovel snow all winter long is enough to drive many people to move to Florida! It's a smart move if you are not in good shape, as shoveling is highly taxing and stressful. According to the American Heart Association, shoveling is the kind of sudden exertion that can put some people at an increased risk for a heart attack, as it raises blood pressure. Shoveling is extremely strenuous even for those who are fit, so be sensible and go slow. This is not the time to be a weekend warrior and put your health and back at risk.

❶ Make sure to warm your body up with five to ten minutes of light cardio exercise (like walking), and do the seven stretches if you can before you go outside to shovel. If not, stretch afterward. Remember, this type of chore can put tremendous strain on your back, so you really should consider stretching beforehand, as it's extremely important to be warm and loose before you tackle the snow you need to clear. But if your time is limited, at least try to stretch afterward.

❷ Whatever kind of snow shovel you choose—whether it has a curved or straight handle—make sure it is the right size for your height. It should be long enough so that you're not bending over just to scoop. Consider using a smaller shovel with a plastic blade. You won't be able to shovel as much per load, but it will weigh less, which can reduce the strain on your back. Wear thick gloves to keep your hands warm and dry, as they also provide a better grip.

❸ Always contract your abdominals with each scoop. Concentrate on pushing the snow out of the way rather than scooping all of it up. Keep your feet shoulder-width apart and bend at the knees when pushing the snow. Never lift the shovel if your knees are not bent—the power should come from your legs, not your back. Keep the shovel close to your body.

❹ When getting the snow off the shovel, bend your legs and contract your abdominals. Do not bend from your waist with your legs straight. Walk over to the area where you are dumping the snow so that you are not leaning over and throwing the snow. Avoid twisting your back when turning your body, and make sure you pivot your foot first. Keep your loads light.

5 Do not hold your breath!

6 Take lots of breaks, and stay hydrated with water. You can do some light stretches during one of your breaks.

7 If you feel any twinges or pain in your joints or muscles, stop immediately and rest. If you feel any tightness in your chest or shortness of breath, stop and seek medical attention.

8 Try to stretch afterward. The Hamstring Wall or Floor Stretch, Knees to Chest Stretch, Spinal Stretch, Piriformis Stretch, Hip Flexors Stretch, Quadriceps Standing or Lying-Down Stretch and Total Back Stretch are all recommended.

9 Try not to let the snow pile up. The earlier you start shoveling, the easier it is to do. And if you have a tendency toward back pain, try to hire someone in the neighborhood to shovel and spare you this task, if at all possible. If you talk to your neighbors about your back, you may be surprised how many people share your pain. You may be able to pool your resources to help each other.

Raking Leaves

Raking is a great way to firm up your arms and shoulders, but it can be very tough on your back, especially if you don't do this kind of sweeping motion regularly.

1 Before you pick up the rake, be sure to warm up and then do the seven stretches. You can do the stretches after you've finished raking, too.

2 Keep your abdominals contracted, and use a rake with a long handle and wide bottom that's not too heavy. Try to alternate arms. This can be tough. You'll see how much stronger your dominant arm is when you switch to the other one—but doing so will give your less utilized muscles a chance to get stronger.

3 When bagging leaves, remember to bend your knees, contract your abdominals and breathe!

4 Do the seven stretches, as they will protect your back and lessen soreness.

Mowing the Lawn

We're not surprised that there are so many accidents involving lawn mowers, as people tend to think of them as a benign contraption to cut the grass, instead of as a heavy, dangerous, vibrating piece of equipment. Worse, it's a heavy piece of equipment you need to push. And if you're like most people, you'll lean forward when pushing and then move backward, off balance, when yanking the mower toward you. These are unnatural positions that put pressure on your back.

1 Before you start, make sure the lawn mower's handle is the correct height. You can find handle extenders at hardware stores or online, and they're easy to attach. Try out the mowers in the garden-supply store, and make sure you don't have to reach too high (if you're short) or hunch over (if you're tall).

2 Always use both hands when mowing, and especially when turning. It's sometimes tempting to only use one hand, but this will easily throw you off balance.

3 It's less stressful for your back to push a mower than to pull it back. Try to avoid pulling it back whenever possible, and never use only one hand if you do pull it back.

4 When turning a lawn mower, go for a wide arc rather than a twisting turn. Keep your feet out of the way of the blades. Safety first!

5 Keep your abdominals contracted when mowing.

6 If you have to bag up the grass, remember to bend your knees, contract your abdominals and breathe!

Gardening

Gardening can be a terrific stress reducer, can make your property look sensational, can feed your family and can improve the environment. But gardening can be very hard on your back, as you'll rarely be upright. Instead, you'll be bending, digging, planting and pulling out those pesky weeds that seemingly sprout up overnight. You can still enjoy your garden if you follow these tips. Be conscious of your posture, and remember to breathe normally.

TIP: Raised gardens and wall or window boxes not only look nice but spare you the extra bending.

TIP: Plan ahead, and try not to do too much in one day. Don't do one chore (like planting or weeding) for a long period and then move on to the next. You don't want to lose track of the time and get stiff. Mix it up whenever possible.

TIP: Wear gardening gloves with a textured grip. They allow you to get your hands dirty, but more important, they help you grip tools and weeds, so you can concentrate on your tasks without slipping or losing your balance.

TIP: When planting, it might be easier to pat down the dirt with your foot instead of your hands, whether you are sitting or standing.

❶ To reduce strain on your back, always contract your abdominals when bending over or pulling. Never bend with straight legs; always squat and keep your knees bent.

❷ Place a cushion or towel under your knees when kneeling to plant. (Gardening catalogues have lots of great cushions and other items you might not have thought of.) Or you can sit on a bucket, a stool or a cushion—whatever is comfortable, as long as you aren't leaning forward too much. Keep your feet spread apart. Make sure whatever you're working on is close to you so you don't have to reach.

❸ If sitting is uncomfortable, get a gardening cushion and weed or plant while on your hands and knees. Be sure to keep your abdominals contracted, and change position every so often.

❹ Using lightweight hand tools while in a seated or kneeling position might be more comfortable for you. Some people prefer to use long-handled tools and do most of their weeding and cultivating from a standing position, but if you do, follow the advice given in the section on Shoveling Snow on p. 115. If you do use tools with long handles, they should be as lightweight as possible.

❺ When weeding, get as close to the beds as possible. Before you start to yank, brace yourself on the ground with your nondominant hand. One hand firmly on the ground will provide a surprisingly large amount of support for your back. If the weeds are deeply entrenched, don't yank. Use your hand cultivator to loosen the roots first. Then sit down and get as close to the weeds as possible. With your legs apart, dig your heels into the ground, your toes pointing up, bend your knees slightly, and then shift the pressure down onto your heels while using both hands to pull. Make sure your abdominals are contracted. It really is easier to weed this way than from a standing position.

❻ Whenever possible, change positions. Take breaks often. If you're down on the ground, stand up and move around for a minute.

❼ Stretch when you can. You can even place a blanket, towel or drop cloth on a level, dry patch of ground and do as many of the seven stretches as you like, bearing in mind that the Total Back Stretch might be challenging to do if there's nothing to hold on to. The more you stretch before and after gardening, the better your back will feel.

CHAPTER 5

MANAGING YOUR BACK PAIN IN BED

A DEEP, RESTFUL, UNTROUBLED SLEEP rejuvenates, refreshes and is always something to look forward to at the end of a long and stressful day. But when going to bed makes your back feel worse, you don't think of sleep as a refuge, but as something to dread. And let's not even get into how back pain can affect your sex life!

For some people, mornings are always the very worst time, as they've spent hours sleeping in one position. Even if they went to bed with the best possible alignment, lying still in one static position for hours—or tossing and turning, with the pillows sometimes ending up on the floor or at the end of the bed—can cause their back to stiffen up overnight, leaving them in agony the minute they reach over to turn off the alarm.

For others, the morning is the only time they experience back pain—which is actually a reaction to the activity of the day before. I often hear from weekend warriors who played a great game of golf or tennis, felt energized and happy, without so much as a twinge of pain, went to bed and had a great night's sleep, and then woke up feeling as if a tractor-trailer had run over them in the middle of the night!

What you'll learn in this chapter is why the morning pain can be so bad, how to get in and out of bed properly and how to have a normal sexual life, when you might have despaired that the intimate moments with your partner would be impossible. Once you start doing your seven stretches, as well as your core exercises, you will be amazed at how much easier it is to sleep better, sleep deeper and get up pain free in the morning.

GETTING IN AND OUT OF BED WHEN YOU'RE IN PAIN

Before you can do anything else, you need to know how to get in and out of bed, as this can be very difficult when you're in a lot of pain. Follow these steps and you will no longer have to worry that these movements will be difficult to manage.

How to Get into Bed

1 Try to do the seven stretches for seven minutes before getting into bed. They will help to loosen up the tight muscles that are putting a strain on your back, so you can relax when you're lying down.

2 Stand with your back toward the bed, then contract your abdominals, and bend your knees slightly, so you look like you're about to squat down. Place one hand on your bed.

3 Slowly lower yourself to the edge of the bed. You should be in a seated position, with your legs hanging over the edge of the bed. Try to place yourself where your hips would be when you're lying down.

4 Lean to your side and go down to your elbow. Then place your other hand in between your elbow and your knees. As your body leans to one side, your knees will bend and your feet will naturally swing up onto the bed.

5 Keep your knees bent as you roll onto your back. Breathe normally.

6 Relax. You made it!

How to Get out of Bed

1 Contract your abdominal muscles, bend your knees and roll onto your side, facing the edge of the bed. Try to get as close to the edge as possible.

2 Use both hands to push yourself up to a seated position. Go slowly, keep your abdominals contracted and breathe normally.

3 Take a moment to rest, if you need to, making sure you are sitting with equal weight on both sides of your buttocks. Your knees are bent, and your feet are resting on the floor. Do not slouch!

4 Place your hands on the sides of your body, and bend your trunk forward from your hips. Slowly start to straighten up.

ROUTINE FOR THE MORNING

We devised this routine for anyone who has back pain first thing in the morning. The objective is to get you up and out of bed with minimal pain. You can do the stretches on the bed (or on the floor, if getting there doesn't hurt too much and you have a cushioned, nonslip mat, such as a yoga mat) as soon as you wake up.

Don't worry if you can't do your normal warm-up from a seated or standing position (such as a short walk). This routine has been specifically designed to be done from a supine (lying down, faceup) position and will warm your muscles before we have you stretch them. But, of course, if you *can*, get up and walk around the house, have your coffee, brush your teeth and take a shower before you start stretching.

The Warm-up Sequence

Before you begin, contract your abdominals just to get into a starting position. This will brace your spine so any further movement won't stress your back. Simply take the pillows away from your head and place them under your knees, if they are not there already. Make sure the blanket is out of the way so it won't get tangled up in your legs.

1. Abdominal Contraction
(With or Without Pillows under Your Knees)

1 Lie on your back, knees bent, hip-width apart. You can place at least two pillows under your knees if you need help keeping your knees bent. Place your arms down by your sides, with your palms facing down. Relax and make sure you are breathing normally.

2 Inhale, and then, on the exhale, contract your abdominals.

3 Hold the contraction for five to ten seconds, and then release. Try to build up to ten seconds.

4 Do this five to ten times.

2. Shoulder Shrug

This releases the tension in your neck and shoulders.

1 Lie on your back, knees bent, shoulder-width apart, feet flat on the floor or the bed, arms by your sides.

2 Inhale, and then, on the exhale, contract your abdominals.

3 Inhale, and bring your shoulders up to your ears. You will be contracting your upper back muscles. Exhale, and then release your upper back muscles and return to the starting position.

4 Do this five times.

3. Pelvic Tilt

1 Lie on your back, knees bent, hip-width apart. Place your arms down by your sides, your palms facing down. Relax and make sure you are breathing normally. Remove any pillows, as this warm-up will be easier without them.

2 Inhale, and then, on the exhale, contract your abdominals and tilt your pelvis back gently. This will press your back into the mattress. This is a subtle movement.

3 Hold the contraction and position for three to five seconds, and then release slowly.

4 Do this ten times.

4. Abdominal Contraction with Foot Up

1 Lie on your back, knees bent, feet flat, arms at your sides, palms face-down. Relax and make sure you are breathing normally.

2 Inhale, and then, on the exhale, contract your abdominals and hold the contraction while lifting your right foot one to two inches up. Then lower your right foot and lift your left foot up.

3 Do this ten times.

4 Do two sets.

5. Abdominal Contraction with Knee Up

1 Lie on your back, knees bent, feet flat, arms at your sides, palms face-down. Relax and make sure you are breathing normally.

2 Inhale, and then, on the exhale, contract your abdominals and hold the contraction while raising your right knee up. Then lower your right knee and raise your left knee up.

3 Do this ten times.

4 Do two sets.

6. Single Knee to Chest

1 Lie on your back, knees bent, and place your hands on top of your thighs.

2 Inhale, and then, on the exhale, contract your abdominals.

3 Simultaneously extend your left knee out to a straight leg and extend your right arm out behind you, then repeat extending your right knee and left arm.

4 Do this ten times with each leg.

5 Do two sets.

The Stretching Sequence

Refer to the stretches on pp. 45–54 in Chapter 2. Do them on the bed in this order.

❶ Hamstring Floor Stretch (if you need assistance, use a towel, belt or pillowcase, prepare the night before).

❷ Knees to Chest Stretch

❸ Spinal Stretch

❹ Piriformis Stretch

❺ Hip Flexors Stretch (using the bed for support)

❻ Quadriceps Lying-Down Stretch

❼ Total Back Stretch (using the edge of the bed for support)

STRETCHING ROUTINE FOR THE EVENING

One of the best things you can do for your back is the seven stretches for seven minutes right before bed. This will automatically loosen up your tight, aching muscles, which might keep you up or wake you up. And this routine is a much safer alternative than sleep medication to help you fall asleep when in pain.

❶ Hamstring Wall or Floor Stretch

❷ Knees to Chest Stretch

❸ Spinal Stretch

❹ Piriformis Stretch

❺ Hip Flexors Stretch

❻ Quadriceps Lying-Down or Standing Stretch

❼ Total Back Stretch

SLEEPING POSITIONS
AND YOUR BED

Sleeping with these adjustments helps to minimize and in some cases eliminate pain when you get up in the morning.

Back Sleepers

Place one or two flat pillows under your head and two pillows under your knees. Try to keep your arms at your sides. It may be hard to keep the pillows from moving, so try putting the knee pillows under your sheet.

Side Sleepers

Once you are on your side, place one or two pillows under your head and one pillow between your knees. You will be in a fetal position.

Stomach Sleepers

If you must sleep on your stomach, here's how you can try to stay in alignment: place a flat pillow under your upper chest and rest your head to either side. Try to sleep with your hands and elbows on either side of your body, with your hands up near your face, with or without flat pillows underneath them. You may want to bend one leg and place a flat pillow under it.

How to Use a Nest of Pillows for Extra Comfort in Bed

Many people who suffer from back pain worry about how they'll feel when they travel overnight, as they often have no control over the comfort of the bed or the pillows in the places they'll be visiting.

One easy way to alleviate these worries is with this nifty nesting technique. You can make a comfortable nest of pillows on any bed, with pillows of any size or firmness, and it will always work. If there aren't enough pillows in the room, you can try using rolled-up throw pillows, towels or blankets.

All you need to do is place one or two pillows under your head and knees, then one under each arm. Make sure your neck is not strained. You might need to experiment with different pillows to find the perfect balance. Once you do, you will be shocked at how unbelievably comfortable this nest is, and how much stress is taken off your back. (Actually, one of the reasons people often like adjustable hospital beds is that they can elevate the lower half, raising their knees and hips and taking the stress off their lower back, which is essentially what the nest of pillows does!) Your weight will remain evenly distributed when you're sleeping; the position of the pillows will prevent you from tossing and turning too much on the bed.

What Kind of Mattress Is Right for My Aching Back?

When shopping for a mattress, think about a slightly different version of what Goldilocks said. "That one might be too hard and that one might be too soft, but *this* one is just right for me."

One of the concepts in ergonomics is anthropometry, which deals with body type (such as ectomorphic, characterized by a lean, slightly muscular body; or endomorphic, characterized by a rounder, less muscular body), weight, height and limb length. Each person has his or her own unique anthropometric measurements—which means that each person wants a different design for beds or other furniture—one that provides maximum comfort for his or her body.

We've found that most people with back pain prefer a mattress that is medium firm, but like everything else, it all comes down to taste and personal comfort. Some people also prefer a platform bed, as that gives firm support to a mattress only, without the springiness of a box spring. However, for those with lower back pain, in general, firm to very firm mattresses are usually preferred from a physiological and kinesiological point of view. The reason is simple: soft beds provide much less support, and your muscles have to work harder to maintain a specific posture or stay in alignment. Another important point is that the softer the mattress, the harder it usually is to get up from it; you automatically sink down when you press down on it.

Mattresses are one item in the house that you really need to take your time testing, in person. Don't buy one when you are in a rush. Wear comfortable clothes and flat shoes, and lie down for as long as you need to on the sample beds. Make sure you lie in your favorite position. Don't fall for the salesperson's hype, as sometimes less expensive mattresses are better for you than expensive, pillowy soft ones. Be sure to rotate the mattress regularly—and it goes without saying that if your back is aching, have someone else do this for you. Mattresses are heavy and unwieldy.

A consumer tip: there are often mattresses on sale online at a great discount. But you should never buy a mattress online unless you are absolutely sure you have already tested that model and feel comfortable on it. Returning a mattress is never easy.

BACK PAIN AND SEX
What about Sex?

Sally sat in my office, and her eyes filled with tears. "This is so embarrassing, but I don't know what to do," she told me. "My back hurts so much that when my husband thought I was moaning with pleasure, I was actually groaning in pain. I couldn't find any position that didn't hurt, but I didn't want to let him know, because it's hard enough for him to put up with me being in pain and irritable all the time as it is. Can you help me?"

I had heard questions like Sally's many times before. I can always tell when my patients have these very specific questions on their minds, as they blush or fidget, and when I see the embarrassed look on their face, I try my best to put them at ease. It can be very difficult to bring up such a personal topic, although you certainly shouldn't be ashamed to talk about it. It is, however, an especially difficult and delicate topic.

Unfortunately, back pain and sex are rarely discussed by the media or by experts, who could give helpful information to those who deserve answers with compassion and understanding.

If you think about it, though, the physical movements that comprise the lovemaking process are those that can put your back at risk. And when you're in the throes of passion, your back is likely the last thing you're thinking about—unless the pain suddenly becomes unbearable.

So I explain to my patients that, yes, they can have sex when their back is hurting, and that there is no one perfect position, so the best thing to do is try whatever position is the most comfortable for them. Having back pain now does not mean that you can't have pleasurable and pain-free sex in the future.

The Psychological Impact of Back Pain on Your Intimate Life

Sex is one of the great pleasures of adult life, and it is a wonderful way to be intimate with your partner and relieve the stress of the day. It is supposed to be a pleasurable activity and something to look forward to with happiness and anticipation. It's something that can always bring you closer to your partner, and it provides that essential emotional connection, but that is much more difficult to find once you are thinking of sex as a chore because you fear that it will lead to back pain.

Any kind of chronic pain can decrease your sex drive, especially when you don't feel confident or attractive. It can also decrease your ability to have pleasurable sex because you fear that it will bring on your pain—or if your partner is the one in pain, you may be afraid to hurt him or her. And if you have been prescribed potent pain medications, these may have side effects that diminish your sexual drive or your ability to perform.

Back pain can definitely change the dynamics of a couple's sexual relationship, and not for the better. I've had patients who've told me that they felt as if their back pain had changed their personality in bed—they were focusing on the pain, not the pleasure. Or if the situation was manageable in the moment, they were still worried that the pain would arrive with a vengeance a few hours later. One patient broke down in tears when she told me that her favorite part of sex wasn't the act itself, but the cuddling and intimate sharing afterward—but she was unable to do that any longer, because if her husband so much as laid an arm or leg on her body, her back would fairly radiate with pain.

I've also had patients who feel terribly guilty because their back pain prevents them from pleasuring their partner the way they *want* to but can't. Others suffer in silence, embarrassed and frustrated that their body is letting them down, and they often blame themselves for something that is certainly *not* their fault. Some of my male patients have discussed how their back pain gets right to the heart of how they feel about their potency as a man. They might not be able to lift the groceries or mow the lawn—and if their sexual performance suffers, this can lead to a lot of depression and suppressed anger.

When back pain is still a regular part of your life—which should change once you incorporate the stretches and core exercises you read about in Chapters 2 and 3 into your daily routine—conversation about intimate issues can be challenging, but it is essential for you to trust your partner and be able to talk openly about fears and insecurities. If you can't talk openly, many misunderstandings and miscommunication can arise, further compounding the problem and intensifying the shame, blame and disappointment. This can take all the fun and anticipation out of sex, which is an essential component of any healthy relationship.

Andrew and Laura's Story

Andrew and Laura were newlyweds in their mid-thirties. They both had demanding careers that necessitated a lot of traveling, which also meant a lot of sitting and pulling luggage, and their hectic schedules meant they didn't have much time for stretching and exercising. (Of course, they also didn't know that it takes only seven minutes to stretch and not much more to work your core, and that these stretches and exercises can be done anywhere, even in a hotel room.) Their only bonding time was at night, but that was out of the question when they were both on the road, so their intimate evenings together were something they both looked forward to with eager anticipation.

Andrew made an appointment to see me after he had an episode of pain that was taking longer than usual to heal. He told me that he had been suffering from lower back pain for many years, but had always been able to manage it with pain medication. But since the medication knocked him out for the night, he really didn't want to take it any longer, as he would much rather be awake in bed with his beloved wife than falling asleep due to a narcotic.

Andrew confided that he was truly in love with Laura and knew how lucky he was. He had been a bachelor for many years and hadn't had much success with women, and he wanted to please Laura as much as possible. He was ecstatic that Laura had a healthy appetite for sex, but much less ecstatic that her wonderful enthusiasm in bed often put him in positions that compromised his back. He joked that this was a very nice problem to have, but he was feeling like a failure because when the pain was severe, he made excuses to avoid sex, and this was starting to put a strain on their marriage. Laura was beginning to worry that Andrew wasn't as attracted to her, when in fact the truth was much simpler. Andrew had been so ashamed about his back pain and had never told her about it for fear that she would think he was weak or faking it. Now the situation was getting worse, and he had to do something about it.

Andrew managed to tell me that the only position that he could manage during their lovemaking sessions was lying on his back, with his wife straddling him, but even that was becoming a big problem, as the pain in his lower back sometimes radiated down his leg and even affected his pelvis, and he couldn't bear the thought of any kind of movement while he was lying down. He found himself almost a passive participant in bed, as Laura had to do most of the "work." She didn't mind, because this role often gave her great pleasure, but she still felt that he was distant. She couldn't help but wonder what was going on, and that made it difficult to concentrate on the fun and joy of being with her husband.

After a particularly serious bout of pain, Andrew finally told Laura about his pain, and she lovingly chided him for not telling her sooner. But then the problem became her anxiety about hurting him; it's difficult to let yourself go and think about your own physical needs and desires when you're worried about hurting the spouse you love! That's when Andrew finally arrived in my office, determined to get better.

During our exam, I ruled out any more serious conditions before explaining how the seven stretches worked and how important it was for him to stretch every day and strengthen his core.

Once Andrew followed my instructions, the pain gradually less-
ened and he was able to move around without injuring his back. He
was thrilled, and he and Laura were able to have a second honeymoon,
deepening their love for each other, as they were able to fully express it
emotionally and physically, without fear of pain or discomfort.

Andrew's situation is a common one—after all, intense sexual activity
is like exercise, and for someone with back pain, it needs to be eased
into slowly. And it's easy to get lost in the moment and not have Back
Mindfulness when you are preoccupied! Regular stretching and core
strengthening really can do wonders.

Back Care Sex Tips

As with any other activities you'll read about in this book, you can
follow these tips to ensure that your back will be protected during sex.
Instead of dreading the pain, you'll know that you can manage it—and
you might even feel really great afterward!

1 Do Kegel exercises during the day. These are extremely simple
exercises that involve contracting the muscles around your genitals, holding the contraction, then releasing. (For more specifics,
ask your gynecologist or urologist for advice.) Kegels can help
improve the stability of the pelvis, which is important for our
spine. Furthermore, studies have shown that Kegels can help men
with erectile dysfunction and women with urinary incontinence;
for both, they can also enhance sexual performance.

Because the movements are so miniscule and internal, no one
will ever know that you are doing them, and this means they can
be done anywhere. You can do them while driving, at work, at the
gym, while watching TV with the kids.

2 As with Kegels, get into the habit of contracting your abdominals
whenever possible. The more you do this, the more it will become
second nature to you. And as you know by now, a tremendous
side benefit is stronger muscles and an improved appearance.
Don't forget to breathe!

❸ Stretching can also start the blood flowing to your genitals, which is a good thing for sexual response. A great way to add stretching into your sexual routine is by thinking of it as foreplay. You and your partner can stretch together—that will not only help your back, but also loosen you up before sex.

If you like to cuddle and have sex first thing in the morning, you might have problems if your back tends to be very stiff after a night's sleep. Try to do the seven stretches right before bed. As soon as you wake up, you might want to take a warm shower and do the warm-up and stretches in this chapter.

❹ Remember to breathe and relax during sex! You may not even realize that you're inadvertently holding your breath.

❺ Massaging your partner is a great way to help get loosened up and put you in the mood. Be sure to use proper pillow placement, as described on pp. 128–129, when you do.

❻ Pillows can help with different positions and make lying in bed a lot easier. Again, use the tips on pp. 128–129 for proper pillow placement, and consider using your partner's legs as pillows if that feels comfortable.

❼ If at all possible, consider stretching after sex. This will loosen you up after what can be intense physical activity. Remember, these seven stretches take only seven minutes!

❽ When you exercise, be sure to work your core muscles. A strong core can make for a hot time in the bedroom—the more flexible you are and the stronger you are, the more you are able to assume and sustain different positions.

Positions for Sex that Cause the Least Amount of Stress on Your Back

Even though lovemaking is a marvelous thing, it is still a physical activity that can place stress on your back. When your core is strong and your muscles are used to being stretched, you will enjoy sex more, not only because you will not have to worry about your back, but also because this strength will enhance your pleasure.

For Women with Back Pain

1 If you're on the bottom, lie on your back with or without pillows under your head, bend your knees and hold on to your legs for support while he enters you. (You will be in a straddle position.) Or instead of holding on to yourself for support, place your arms around your partner's back or grab hold of his arms while keeping your knees bent. Holding on to him might give you more control so that he doesn't apply too much body weight on you. Try to contract your abdominals, and keep them contracted the entire time. (If you're like most women, you want to have a flat stomach during the throes of passion—and at all other times. Doing these contractions daily has the double bonus of improving both your figure and your sex life!)

2 Lie on your back, with your partner on his side. Place your bent knees over his pelvic area so he can enter you this way. You can use pillows under your head and lower back for support.

3 Sit on top of your partner when he is flat on his back, either facing him or with your back toward him. Use his legs for support if your back is toward him. This position might feel better as you can hold on to his legs for support. Remember to contract your abdominals, and keep them contracted as much as possible.

4 If you are in a kneeling position, you may want to bend over something height appropriate, and make sure you place pillows under your knees. If you are on all fours, place pillows under your trunk at a height high enough to support you. Remember to contract your abdominals, and keep them contracted as much as possible.

5 Lying flat on your stomach can place a lot of stress on your lower back. But if you do assume this position, try placing pillows under your pelvis or stomach for support.

6 A chair might feel good. See if it is better to face your partner or turn your back toward him. If your back is toward him, you can use the armrest or his legs for support. You might like it if he holds your arms when your back is to him, as this can hold you upright, as long as he doesn't pull your arms back too far. If you face him and the chair is high, you can put pillows or something else under your feet, depending on the chair height.

For Men with Back Pain

❶ Standing behind her while she is on the bed might be hard for you to do if the bed is low, as you will not have great support for your back from this angle. Thrusting while your legs are straight in the missionary position can also place a lot of stress on your lower back. But if this is your pleasure, make sure you contract your abdominals.

❷ If you are on your back, place a pillow under your head and another one under your knees. Your partner can be on top of you, either facing you or with her back toward you. If you can't take the pressure on your legs, then instead of her using your legs for support, hold her arms behind her (she will be more upright).

❸ If you're on top, place pillows under your partner to bring her up closer to you.

❹ If you want to kneel, you can put a pillow under your knees for support.

❺ If you're on a chair, it might be better if your partner has her back to you, as less weight will be placed on your body when her legs rest on the floor.

What If Your Back Seizes Up during or after Sex?

Protection Mode will help you if your back seizes up when you least want it to! Contract your abdominals so that you can move with confidence to a comfortable position, and then read about Protection Mode on pp. 56-61 in Chapter 2.

Try doing the seven stretches on the bed or on the floor, as outlined on pp. 124-126 in this chapter. An anti-inflammatory medication, such as Advil, might also help.

CHAPTER 6

MANAGING YOUR BACK PAIN AT WORK

IF YOU'RE LIKE MANY PEOPLE, your typical workday might start something like this: the alarm goes off at 6 A.M., and as you reach over to hit the button after a night of restless slumber, the first thought in your head is, *Oh, my back is killing me.* Then you get out of bed with a grimace; go downstairs to make coffee; head back upstairs to shower, shave or put on your makeup, and dry your hair; and then go back downstairs and sit at the table or lean over the counter (ouch) to eat and drink your coffee. Then it's back upstairs to wake the kids and brush your teeth, when you wonder again why your back hurts so much when you're leaning over the sink. Then you rush around, taking care of the kids and seeing them off to the school bus before getting into the car with your heavy briefcase at your side. If you're lucky, you have a short commute; if not, you're stuck in traffic, barely able to manage more uncomfortable sitting. And you haven't even gotten to your office yet!

So by the time you arrive at your desk, sit down and check your email, your back is already screaming, yet you have an entire day of work ahead, with all the usual bending over to pick things up or twisting behind you to get that file or talk to a colleague.

Or what if you are a delivery person and you never know exactly how much each package weighs before you pick it up? What if you are a nurse and are on your feet for your entire shift, getting patients out of bed and to the bathroom or helping them bathe or turning them over to check their vital signs? What if you're a firefighter or police officer, loaded down with heavy and cumbersome equipment? Or what if you work in a restaurant, carrying heavy trays in an awkward position? Or what if you are a teacher and you have to bend down to talk to students all day?

Most of us work at jobs that are—believe it or not—backbreakers, although we realize it only when we are in pain. You don't have to be a furniture mover or farmer to spend most of the day engaging your back. If you sit for many hours, you are at risk for back problems. You have to work, you have to sit and you have to sit in the chair and at the workstation that is given to you, so it's no wonder your back is aching at the end of the day.

I know this firsthand, as surgeons often need to hunch over the patients they're working on for hours at a time, and this can put a lot of stress on our neck. It's an occupational hazard, and I often don't realize how little I've moved when I'm concentrating with minute precision on the work at hand. Obviously, remaining in any position for any length of time is not good for anyone's back.

This is a problem that must be addressed—but often isn't—as your back pain is not going to go away on its own, especially if you don't know what to do, and you fear that getting better will either take a huge amount of time or be extremely costly to manage. Unaddressed back pain leads to workplace absenteeism, costs incurred by workmen's compensation and billions of dollars in lost productivity. To say nothing of the suffering endured by those in pain!

Happily, doing the 7-Minute Back Pain Solution can stop the back pain and prevent it from flaring in the future. Armed with Back Mindfulness, you can make so many easy adjustments to your workdays, so that you'll soon be able to concentrate on your work—not on your aching back.

WHAT HAPPENS TO YOUR BACK WHEN YOU SIT?

Because many of us spend long hours at work in a seated position, it's very important to understand what happens to your body when you sit. Contrary to popular belief, being seated is not a great or a natural position for your body, but because many people think it's comfortable, they're completely unaware of the stress put on their back when they sit down.

When you're at home relaxing in your favorite comfortable chair, you're free to get up and move around or put your feet up. Sitting at work, however, is often a lot more stressful because you're tense. You're concentrating, you have countless things demanding your attention, the email is pinging and the phone is ringing, your boss is in a bad mood, and on top of it, you're worried about your deadlines and getting out of the office in time to pick up your kids. You know you can manage the tasks at hand, but what happens to your muscles is they clench up. Then you get tired and you slump, or you lean forward or tilt to one side or place your arms awkwardly on your desk. All these movements can contribute to stress on your lower back.

When you sit, you immediately shift the alignment of your hips to your spine; this alignment is easier to maintain when you're standing or walking. As you learned in Chapter 1, sitting makes your hip flexors and hamstrings tighten up, and your abdominal and gluteal muscles slacken off if they're not engaged. (Really, who thinks to contract their buttocks while seated at work—you've got many other things on your mind!) Sitting also puts a lot of stress on the erector muscles of your back, especially when you lean over to work on a computer or at your desk. This pulls your pelvis out of alignment, which then pulls on your lower back muscles, taking you out of the neutral spine position. If your core muscles are not in shape, sitting can cause significant strain, resulting in lower back pain.

If, on the other hand, your core muscles have been stretched, leaving them flexible and supple, and if they are strong and equally balanced with all the muscles they work synergistically with, you can easily maintain a neutral spine position while seated. Thus Back Mindfulness and core strength keep lower back pain away.

TOP TIPS FOR MANAGING BACK PAIN AT WORK

❶ Start incorporating the seven stretches into your daily routine whenever and wherever possible.

② If you have to sit all day, get up regularly; if you stand all day, sit down regularly. Don't sit for more than twenty minutes without getting up or changing your position. Do your best to get off your office chair and walk around. You can do a few of the stretches when you are on the phone or checking your email. You can always work on contracting your abdominals and keeping them contracted for long stretches.

Believe me, I know how hard it can be to do this—once surgeons start operating, we must finish the procedure, even if our back and neck are aching. You might work at a job that requires tremendous concentration, and you can honestly lose track of the time when you're deeply involved in the work at hand. Just bear in mind that regular breaks lasting a few minutes can prevent days of problems later, if your lower back starts hurting because you stay at your desk all day.

③ Design your workstation as ergonomically as possible. See the section on pp. 150–153 for more details.

④ Be mindful of your back at all times! Be aware of your posture. Don't slump or slouch. Remember to contract those abdominals before you make any movements (twisting, bending down, leaning over, lifting) that can stress your lower back. This means, think of your back first in every situation at work. Once you start doing this, it will quickly become second nature, and you will be amazed at how easy it is to protect your back no matter what you do.

⑤ Use a footrest at your desk, as this keeps your feet in better alignment with your hips and helps keep you in the neutral spine position. If you don't have a footrest, you can use old telephone books, or place a firm pillow atop a weighted box that won't shift around.

⑥ Plan ahead, which is another component of Back Mindfulness. Arrange work-related items on your desk and prepare for the day's tasks before you sit down. If, for example, you need to work with a lot of files, gather all of them before you start. Place them close by, preferably atop your desk, so you don't have to keep bending over or twisting to get them out of a filing cabinet.

7 Never cradle the phone on your neck. If you need to use the phone constantly at work, get a good wireless headset.

8 Use a backpack, and carry it on your back, not on your shoulders! Or opt for a backpack that rolls. See the sidebar Attack of the Killer Backpacks on p. 145 for more information.

9 Wear comfortable shoes or sneakers to get to work, and if possible, keep them on during the day. Women who wear high heels automatically put more stress on their lower back. Either carry dressier shoes to work or keep them in your desk to change into at work, if needed.

10 Feel free to fidget. If you just can't get up from your chair due to a demanding project, go ahead and squirm! Just remember to contract your abdominals and rotate your pelvis forward, then backward. Doing this a few times should release some tightness.

11 Keep moving during the day as much as possible. Use the stairs, if you can manage it. Park your car an extra distance from the office so you have to walk. Instead of eating lunch at your desk, take your back for a walk. Place your printer away from your desk, so you have to get up to retrieve documents. The exercise is great for your body and costs nothing.

12 If your job necessitates standing all day, at least try to shift your weight from side to side and be Back Mindful of your posture. Standing on one foot for a few seconds can help. If you stand behind a counter, place a cushioned mat under your feet for support.

13 When you get home, don't head right for that overstuffed lounger or your inviting bed to take the load off. The very best way to take the load off is by working your core and doing the seven stretches. Not only will this routine help relieve the stress of the day, but it will get you energized for the rest of the evening.

Rest Breaks Aren't Slacking—They're Essential

There are two types of work: static and dynamic. An example of static work is a job done at a computer or at an office desk; an example of dynamic work is that done by carpenters, plumbers, waitstaff, chefs, police officers and delivery people.

One of the biggest difficulties with both types of work is figuring out the appropriate work/rest schedule—what ergonomists call recovery, or rest breaks—that is ideal for your body and back health. For static work, recovery involves movement, such as leaving the computer workstation and walking or stretching. For dynamic work, recovery involves rest.

With static work, local muscles—like those in your lower back—are usually involved, so the recovery should be frequent but not long. This means getting up from your workstation and moving around or stretching for a few minutes.

Conversely, with dynamic work, entire muscle groups are involved. Workers can stay on the job longer, but they need longer periods of recovery, during which their body gets a break from any of the kind of movement usually done at work.

Problems arise, not surprisingly, because there are many variables that affect the work schedule for every occupation. Plus, every worker on the job has many variables affecting his or her own health. For example, a young employee who is active and fit will likely be more determined to go for a short walk regularly during breaks, while someone with diabetes and circulatory problems might want to stay at a desk during breaks because they don't feel great.

Businesses whose managers want a healthy and vibrant workforce allow ample time during the workday for appropriate rest breaks. Smart bosses know that allowing their employees to move around regularly actually increases productivity. Employees become more alert because movement—including stretching—always stimulates blood flow, which is nourishing for your entire body. If your boss isn't enlightened or your office isn't conducive to movement, still try your best to get a move on as much as possible.

Attack of the Killer Backpacks

When the Beatles sang, "Boy, you're gonna carry that weight," I am sure they didn't mean for our children to really carry ridiculously heavy schoolbooks crammed into a backpack they have to lug to and from school every day. According to the American Academy of Orthopaedic Surgeons, the optimal fit for a backpack is two inches above the waist. How many kids do you see with a backpack resting that high on their back? (I've yet to see any!)

The same rule applies to adults, who also tend to carry overloaded backpacks.

Backpack Checklist

1. The backpack should hang no less than two inches above the waist.
2. It should have wide padded straps.
3. Use both straps—not one—to carry the backpack. If one is the choice (perhaps between classes), be sure to switch sides frequently.
4. The heaviest books should be worn closest to the back.
5. When lifting heavy backpacks, always bend at the knees. Use leg power, not your back!
6. The backpack should not weigh more than 20 percent of a child's or teen's body weight.
7. If your child or teen has recurring back pain, get a note from your physician allowing him or her to keep a second set of books at home. Also look for a rolling backpack, although these often have to be carried up and down stairs.

BACK-SAVING ROUTINE IN SEVEN MINUTES OR LESS FOR THE OFFICE

This routine is done from your chair.

1. Abdominal Contraction from Your Chair

1 Sit on a chair with your feet flat on the floor, hip-width apart, your back touching the back of the seat, and your hands on your belly.

2 Inhale, and then, on the exhale, contract your abdominals. Hold the contraction for five to ten seconds, and then release slowly.

3 Do this ten times. You can do more if you like—just be sure not to hold your breath.

2. Pelvic Tilt

1 Sit tall on a chair with your feet flat on the floor, hip-width apart, your back touching the back of the seat, and your hands on your belly. Relax and make sure you are breathing normally.

2 Inhale, and then, on the exhale, contract your abdominals and tilt your pelvis back.

3 Hold the contraction and the position for three to five seconds, and then release slowly.

4 Do this five to ten times.

Northport-East Northport Public Library

The following item(s) were checked out
on 08/30/2022

Title: **The 7-minute back pain solution : 7 simple**
Author: Girasole, Gerard.
Barcode: 30602002598651
Due: **09-27-22**

Title: How civil wars start : and how to stop
Author: Walter, Barbara F., author.
Barcode: 30602003106561
Due: **09-20-22**

Total items checked out: 2

You just saved an estimated $43.95 by
using the library today.

Northport	**East Northport**
151 Laurel Avenue	185 Larkfield Road
Northport, NY 11768	East Northport, NY 11731
631-261-6930	(631) 261-2313

www.nenpl.org

3. Neck Stretch

1 Sit tall on a chair with your feet flat on the floor, hip-width apart, your back touching the back of the seat, and your arms at your sides.

2 Slowly tilt your head toward your right shoulder, then toward your left shoulder, and then drop your chin toward your chest. Hold this position for two to three seconds. Breathe normally and move slowly.

3 Do this two times.

4. Shoulder Shrug

1 Sit tall on a chair with your feet flat on the floor, hip-width apart, your back touching the back of the seat, and your arms at your sides.

2 Inhale, and then, on the exhale, contract your abdominals.

3 Slowly raise your shoulders up toward your ears, hold for a few seconds, and then slowly lower them. It should take three seconds to go up and three seconds to go down.

4 Do this five to ten times.

The next two exercises are not meant to be done in the same session. Pick whichever one is the most comfortable.

5. Seated Twist

1 Sit tall on a chair with your feet flat on the floor, hip-width apart, your back touching the back of the seat, and your arms at your sides.

2 Inhale, and then, on the exhale, contract your abdominals.

3 Cross your left leg over your right leg. Then place both arms over to your left side and slowly twist at your waist so you can look over at your right shoulder.

4 Hold this position for five seconds, and then switch sides, crossing your right leg over your left leg.

5 Do this two times.

6. Piriformis Stretch

1 Sit tall on a chair with your feet flat on the floor, hip-width apart, your back touching the back of the seat.

2 Inhale, and then, on the exhale, contract your abdominals.

3 Cross your right leg over your left leg so that your right ankle is resting on your left thigh.

4 Place your right hand on your right ankle and your left hand on your right knee, and then slowly lower your upper body down toward them. Stop lowering yourself as soon as you feel the stretch in the right piriformis muscle, located on the side of your right hip and buttock. Do not round your back.

5 Hold this position for fifteen seconds, and then switch, this time crossing your left leg over your right leg.

The next three stretches are done standing up.

7. Quadriceps Standing Stretch

1 Stand next to a sturdy piece of furniture, and hold on to it for balance with your left hand.

2 Grasp your right foot (or ankle, if that's easier) with your right hand, and gently pull your leg back and up, with your toes pointing toward your head. Make sure your left knee remains straight.

3 Hold this position for thirty seconds.

4 Switch to your left leg and repeat.

8. Hip Flexor One Cheek Chair Stretch – Variation 2

1 Stand with a sturdy chair on your right side, and then place only your right buttock on the seat. Keep your right leg bent in front of you.

2 Slide your left leg behind you to get a comfortable stretch in the front of your left hip.

3 Hold this position for thirty seconds.

4 Switch sides and repeat.

9. Total Back Stretch

1 Stand next to a sturdy chair, knees bent. Contract your abdominals, and then grasp the chair with both hands, keeping your arms straight. Keep your head level with your shoulders.

2 Hold this position for ten seconds.

3 Stand up straight, place your right hand on your waist and your left arm up over your head, and then side bend to the right. You can use the chair for support if you need to.

4 Hold this position for ten seconds, and then switch sides.

HOW TO SET UP AN ERGONOMIC WORKSTATION FOR YOUR OFFICE

Ergonomics is the science and study of the relationship between each person and his or her environment. It is also all about fitting or matching the job to the worker, rather than forcing the worker to fit into the job. Ideally, you want to work in a place where your body is comfortable and you are able to maintain a neutral spine position, putting the least amount of stress on your lower back (as well as your head, neck and the rest of your body!).

Because no two bodies or backs are alike, everyone will have different requirements for the ideal workstation. This is where problems for workers can instantly arise, as most office furniture and spaces are designed for those of average height, and if you don't fit comfortably, your back can bear the brunt of the stresses put on your body. In addition, many of us can't afford or are not allowed to bring different chairs or desks into our workspace. So you've got to make whatever adjustments you can so that your setup is as ergonomic and back friendly as possible. Luckily, that's not too hard to do.

There are many things you can do that are inexpensive, yet will make a huge difference. For instance, a footrest costs little (or is free, if you use old phone books) yet does wonders for aligning your posture and helping you maintain a neutral spine position. Or a small wrist rest for the hand you use to manipulate the computer mouse may help alleviate carpal tunnel syndrome, or pressure on the median nerve in your wrist, a condition that affects the feeling and movement in your hand. Obviously, carpal tunnel syndrome isn't directly related to lower back pain, but if your wrist and hand hurt, you are likely to tense up. And where does the tension go? Into your shoulders, through your neck and down to your lower back.

Workstations for Your Office That Will Not Stress Your Back

As you know by now, when you sit for a living, your posture puts you out of alignment, repetitive tasks can lead to muscle fatigue and stress can increase tightness and muscle tension. Add to this the most common mistakes made at your desk—sitting for twenty or thirty minutes in the same position and hunching over your desk—and back pain can result. Remember, small changes can have big benefits!

For even more details about ergonomics at work, an excellent source of information is the National Institutes of Health website, www.ors.od.nih.gov. The NIH's Office of Research Services, Division of Occupational Health and Safety, has many lists with specific information for different workplace situations.

Setting Up Your Workstation

Whatever your industry or occupation, the most important factor when it comes to preventing back pain is workstation adjustability. Because everyone has different anthropometric measurements (body type, height, weight and limb length), in an ideal work world, every employee would be allowed to adjust his or her workstation to achieve a perfect fit. No two backs are alike, so why should office equipment or furniture be one-size-fits-all?

Another important consideration when setting up your workstation is symmetry, using both the right and left sides of your body. A concept ergonomists call "exposure/dose/health effect" is critical for the workplace. The more a worker uses a particular limb (such as your right arm and shoulder), the more adverse the health effect usually is. For example, right-sided computer mouse users usually become symptomatic first on their right side. In chronic conditions, the left side will eventually become symptomatic due to, in part, systemic inflammation and to the mouse user favoring the right side. With back pain, this means that if your right side is hurting and you overcompensate by using more of your left side, over time the left side will start hurting as well.

Strive to apply Back Mindfulness when you are seated at your workstation, and try not to favor one side over the other. One way to do this if you work on a computer is to train your nondominant hand to use the computer mouse; since you normally use this hand much less than the other, engaging it regularly will prevent you from overusing your dominant hand.

Sitting at Your Desk Checklist

❶ Sit as close to your desk as possible.

❷ Your buttocks should be as far back on the seat as possible, with your back supported by the back of the chair.

❸ Sit up straight, with your shoulders back. Don't slouch or hunch forward, as this puts pressure on your discs.

❹ Shift around so you distribute your body weight evenly.

❺ Your knees should be even with or slightly higher than your hips. A footstool is a great aid to correct positioning.

❻ If you don't use a footstool, your feet should be flat on the floor. Try not to cross your legs, but if you do, be sure to switch positions frequently.

❼ Your monitor should be at eye level. If it isn't (and few are), place some heavy, sturdy, thick books underneath the monitor to raise it up. This is extremely important, because if you look down at a screen all day, you place a lot of stress on your cervical spine. Your monitor should also be at arm's length from you. Tilt the screen back ten to twenty degrees to avoid glare.

❽ If you use a laptop, connect it to an eye-level monitor. If you can't, place something under it to elevate it. If you use it on your lap, elevate it and make sure your knees are in line with your hips, as this will make you less likely to slouch or lean forward.

9 If your desk chair has wheels and you have to turn or reach back for something, always contract your abdominals first and use your feet to turn your whole body—not just your waist! If there are no wheels, you can turn with your waist as long as you contract your abdominals when doing so.

10 If your chair has a rounded back or is not particularly comfortable or supportive, place a small rolled-up towel, a firm pillow from home or a lumbar cushion in the space between your lower back and the chair. This provides additional support to your lower back because it anchors you upright and neutralizes the natural curve (or lordosis) of your back, as well as giving support to the muscles around your spine. It also makes you less likely to slump or slouch.

11 Rest your elbows on the armrests of your chair or on your desk when possible (and without hunching). Keep your shoulders relaxed.

12 Don't cradle the phone between your shoulder and ear. Use a headset.

13 If you can work from a standing position, try getting a stand-up desk. It's a real back saver.

14 Get up from your desk while you're talking on the phone. It's a great way to do some moving while at work.

15 Be sure to get up and stretch!

The Best Work Chair for Your Back

1. Your chair should be fully adjustable and maximally padded.

2. It should roll on casters and have a five-point base, as this helps distribute your weight and allows for ease of movement.

3. Armrests can help if you have lower back pain, but they can be an issue for computer work, since if they aren't designed well, they

can prevent you from getting close enough to the keyboard and mouse. This can adversely affect your posture. Look for a chair with adjustable armrests that are firmly padded and wide, as the armrest supports the elbow and forearm. This will help take some of the stress off your lower back and neck.

Using a Stand-up Desk

Jonathan is a salesman and spends most of his workday either sitting in his car, sitting at his desk or sitting on airplanes. His back pain went away once he started doing the seven stretches and core exercises—and when he replaced his old work desk with a stand-up desk. He found that he didn't need to get up every twenty minutes or so, as he was already up, and he was able to move around much more when he was on the phone.

A stand-up desk might not be an option for your office, but if it is, it might be worthwhile to give one a try. "Basically," Jonathan said, "that desk saved my life."

How One Hairdresser Helped Ease His Aching Back

Those who work in any service profession are at risk for back problems, as their jobs involve a lot of twisting, bending, leaning-over and lifting motions, they're on their feet all day, their clients are sometimes demanding and their hours are sometimes long, and so it's very difficult to incorporate Back Mindfulness into the tasks at hand.

Hairdressers might not use heavy equipment, but their jobs can be backbreaking: they spend their days wielding scissors and brushes over heads of varying heights, bending over, walking around and stooping over to wash hair in a sink. So when Cara's hairdresser, Michael, told her that his back was killing him after only the third client of the day, she helped him relieve some of the stress with these tips. These will work for anyone who has a similar occupation:

- Wear comfortable shoes.

- Wear a smock or an apron with large, deep pockets for lightweight items. Or use a tool belt as long as your tools are very lightweight and will not pull down on your lower back or hips.

- Use a wheeled trolley to keep all your most used equipment handy, as this will prevent unnecessary twisting.

- Sit and roll around on a sturdy wheeled stool whenever it's possible. Alternate between sitting and standing to incorporate recovery periods.

Managing Your Back Pain in a Classroom

Cara has a friend whose daughter is a fifth grader and is very tall for her age. She is already suffering from neck aches and backaches because the desks and chairs at her school are too small for her. As they grow older, many students who are very short or very tall have trouble with the uncomfortable seating at their school or university. This can become a real problem, as it is almost impossible for them to bring their own ergonomically designed furniture to a classroom or library, and if they are in a large lecture hall, it can be difficult to get up and stretch or leave during the middle of a class if their back starts to hurt. So here are some tips to help you or your children:

- Back Mindfulness will help. Be aware of your posture and your surroundings, and try to sit up as straight as you can. Keep your abdominal muscles engaged as much as possible.

- Bring your own lumbar support to class. This can be a firm pillow or a cushion placed comfortably at the small of your back. Or sit on a firm pillow or cushion, if you prefer.

- Use your backpack or even your books to elevate your feet. If your backpack or books aren't handy, you can take your shoes off and place your feet atop them.

- If possible, try to work at long tables rather than desks/chairs with a fixed arm on one side, as the latter constrains the body and promotes non-neutral spine and elbow positions.

- Wear flat, comfortable shoes.
- One physician I know suffered from chronic back pain during her first year of medical school. Fortunately, her professors understood and allowed her to stand up in the back of the classroom when she needed to. It can't hurt to talk to your teachers or professors about your back. Ask your own physician for a medical note explaining the situation, and you might be able to take your classes without worrying about your back pain.

CHAPTER 7

MANAGING YOUR BACK PAIN ON THE ROAD

Picture this: during a long drive on a Connecticut interstate, a young mom with two toddlers strapped into the car seats in the back hit a bad traffic jam. Naturally, as soon as the cars were barely creeping along, her three-year-old daughter dropped her pacifier and started to scream. What did this mom do? What every already tense and frazzled mom of a screaming kid in the middle of traffic would do—she put her car in park, then leaned over and twisted down to find the pacifier.

That's all it took for the pain to strike. One simple, quick twist.

Drivers often get stuck in traffic for long periods, in cars with seats that might not be very comfortable. Or they need to travel long distances in their cars, or on trains, buses and airplanes, which can wreak havoc on their back and overall health, too. If you have lower back pain, the thought of sitting for an extended period of time in a car—and in a static position guaranteed to increase the stress on your lower back, neck and shoulders—is enough to keep you home all day.

Once you apply Back Mindfulness when you're on the road, however, you can avoid the kind of back pain this mom endured. Thinking of how to protect your back—coupled with the flexibility you'll get from the seven stretches, as well as the core strength you'll get from the core exercises—will make your time on the road far less stressful.

DRIVING AND LOWER BACK PAIN

As you doubtless know already, driving and lower back pain can be a debilitating and uneasy partnership. For most Americans, driving is a daily inevitability, and unlike time spent in an office, where you can get up and move around, once you're in a car and en route to your destination, you can't get up and out unless you pull over and stop, which isn't always possible or safe. It's also hard to redistribute your weight when you're stuck in the same position for what can be a long period of time. This can cause pressure, discomfort, pain and fatigue.

What Sitting in a Car Does to Your Lower Back

Sitting in a car is not the same as sitting in a chair, primarily because you are in motion. This subjects your body to different physical forces: you're moving forward or backward; you turn to see who's passing you; the car moves at varying speeds; and you must keep your foot on the gas pedal or the brake, so you can't use it to help support or stabilize your back. In addition, if you're a good driver, you are always scanning the horizon and the mirror for cars nearby. You are alert and focused— but if there are problems on the road, whether from other drivers, traffic, weather or distractions in the car (if your children are vocal!), you are going to be tensed up and stressed.

Driving can also be made worse for those with back pain because the seats are often uncomfortable. As you know already, sitting stresses your back muscles, makes your hip flexors and hamstrings tighten up, and makes your abdominal and gluteal muscles slacken off if they're not engaged. This pulls your pelvis out of alignment, tugging on your lower back muscles and taking you out of the neutral spine position. If your core muscles are weak, this can lead to significant strain, which can cause lower back pain.

In addition, your driving position or posture affects what ergonomists call the kinematic chain, in which each joint is connected to the joint above and below. For example, if your shoulder hurts, the joints on the kinematic chain are located in your neck and upper back, as well as your elbow. For your lower back, the joints to watch out for are those in your pelvic area and your thoracic spine.

TOP TIPS FOR MANAGING
BACK PAIN WHILE DRIVING

1 Before even getting into the car, start your day off right. If you can't exercise before going to work, warm up for ten minutes, do some core exercises and finish with the seven stretches. If you don't have time for all the core exercises, do a couple in the morning and then do some when you get home. This will definitely take the edge off your commute.

2 As with your office chair, adjustability is key. This can be very difficult if you already own a car with an uncomfortable seat or if you are renting one. Be sure to make seat comfort a priority when getting a new car.

Ideally, your driver's seat is adjustable forward and backward. For actual sitting postures, the pelvic angle should be greater than 95 degrees, with a recommended sitting angle between 95 and 115 degrees. Your buttocks should be touching the back of the seat so there is no slouching. This is to reduce compression forces on the lower back. An electronic tilt up and down can help, as can an adjustable lumbar support and neck rest built into the backrest.

If you need additional lumbar support, place a small rolled-up towel, a firm pillow or a lumbar cushion designed for drivers in the space between your lower back and the seat. This provides additional support to your lower back because it anchors you upright and neutralizes the natural curve (or lordosis) of your back, as well as giving support to the muscles around your spine.

3 The steering wheel should not be too far from or too close to your body. Keep it level so your shoulders are relaxed. Look for one that is adjustable for your height and moves up and down or forward and back for your arm comfort.

4 Contract your abdominal muscles as much as possible while driving, as this can help brace you when you go over bumps or make turns. Contract them when turning back to gauge traffic or park, too.

⑤ Always keep your left leg bent slightly and relaxed.

⑥ Make sure your back pockets are empty, as sitting on your phone or wallet can aggravate your back.

⑦ Make slight adjustments when on long drives, such as moving the seat up or down slightly, and then go back to the original position. Movement helps with stiffness.

⑧ Seat heaters are a great idea, as heat can help ease and relax tight and tense muscles. If your drive is long, alternate turning the heat on and off.

⑨ When looking back, contract your abdominals and breathe normally, and then place your right hand on the passenger headrest for support. This way you won't hurt your lower back when turning your body.

⑩ Recovery is extremely important when driving. Try to take frequent rest breaks, at least once every forty minutes, if at all possible. Get out of the car and do some stretching!

Getting into the Car

❶ Don't rush! Contract your abdominals; then open the car door. If you have a tendency to slouch when you do this, slightly bend your knees when opening the door.

❷ Hold on to the top of the door with your left hand, and then place your right hand on the top of the steering wheel. Or place your left hand on the side of the car.

❸ Place your right leg into the car. Using the steering wheel for support, bend your knees and squat down, putting your right buttock on the seat first and then the left.

❹ Remember to breathe.

Getting out of the Car

❶ Keep your hands free. You can get your bag(s) later.

❷ Place your right hand on the steering wheel, contract your abdominals, and then slowly open the door with your left hand.

❸ Place both hands on the steering wheel for support, and slowly turn your knees and body to face the outside.

❹ Place your feet outside the car. While seated on the edge of the seat, place your hands on the sides of your body, contract your abdominals and push up with your hands. Lean slightly forward, and rise to a standing position.

Loading and Unloading the Trunk

The strength for these loading and unloading maneuvers should come from your arms and legs, not your back. The seemingly simple act of unloading the car is notorious for causing a great deal of back pain, particularly for those who have already sat for an extended period in the car, unable to get up and walk or stretch. They then go from a stressful static position to an unusual motion—lean over the trunk before lifting. It is especially important to use Back Mindfulness when getting anywhere near your trunk!

❶ Think about using a chair or a stool when you load or unload. Keep one handy in the garage just in case, and see if using it helps your back. You don't use it as a seat, but as an elevated support for whatever items you're lifting. You place them on the chair or stool, instead of carrying them directly from the car to the house, or vice versa. This additional step adds but a few seconds to the process. You can also place one foot on the bottom rung of a stool for additional support if you need it, as you would for any leaning-over task.

❷ When you are loading, try to place items as close to the edge of the trunk as possible, so you don't have that far to reach when unloading.

❸ Have the item at chest height before placing it in the trunk.

❹ Contract your abdominals, face the trunk and stand as close to it as you can. Leaning against the car will support you better. Remember to breathe normally.

5 Make sure your feet are shoulder-width apart; then squat down gently for loading, allowing your knees to touch the car for support. Or you can get into a straddle position, which is a squat with your feet wider than shoulder-width apart and your toes pointed out. This position will allow you to get as close to the trunk as possible.

6 Lower the item and slowly rise up. When you're about to turn away from the car, make sure you turn foot first and have your body follow.

7 You can also use a footstool when loading the car. Place one foot on the stool, contract your abdominals, breathe normally, and then squat down slightly and place the item in the trunk.

8 Another alternative is to load from your side. Stand with your side to the trunk, making sure that you are touching the car with your body so you can use it for support. Contract your abdominals, breathe normally, go into a slight squat, and then turn your upper body toward the inside of the trunk and place the item down. Use the edge of the car for support, and then slowly rise up.

9 When unloading the car, reverse the above steps. Make sure you get out and walk around or stretch for a few minutes before you unload the trunk, especially after a long trip.

Tips for Commuters on Mass Transit

1. Make sure that when you are sitting in your seat, you position yourself correctly. Your buttocks should be as close to the back of your seat as possible, and your shoulders should be back. Keep your arms relaxed.

2. Lumbar supports are helpful, as you know. Keep a small, firm pillow or a towel in your bag, and place it against the small of your back, or higher up, if this feels better, making sure your buttocks touch the back of the seat comfortably. If your seat has armrests,

use them. If you have to cross your legs, switch positions every few minutes.

3. A footrest is ideal to get your knees in line with your hips, but that's probably not going to be an option. If you're on a train or bus, try using your briefcase as a footrest, or take your shoes off, if you like, and rest your feet on top. You can also slip your feet out of your shoes to rest them on top of the shoes themselves; this will elevate your feet, legs and hips slightly. You can rest your feet on sturdy packages, or put the packages under your arms and lean on them for support.

4. If you have to stand on a bus or a train or in a subway car, place your bag or briefcase between your feet, which will free up your hands for better gripping. If you have a purse, try to place it so it hangs in front of you. Place both hands on a pole, if possible, with one hand slightly higher than the other. Switch the position of your hands from time to time. Try to contract your abdominals when you're coming to a stop. Make sure to bend slightly at your knees, contract your abdominals and breathe when picking up your bag or briefcase.

LONG-DISTANCE TRAVEL AND YOUR LUGGAGE

We have two words for you about getting ready for a long-distance trip: pack light!

Long-distance travel can be very stressful, so remember to protect your back, because no one else will. Travel can definitely be a workout, and you need to use Back Mindfulness to prepare accordingly. Get to the airport or train/bus station early so you're not rushing, which will make you tense and add to the stress. Remember to contract your abdominals when pushing, pulling or lifting your bags. The last thing you want to do is injure your back on the way to the airport or train/bus station.

Packing Your Luggage

1 Place everything you want to take on the bed or on a firm table, and then put three-quarters of it back, because you're not going to need it or wear it. Be ruthless. Everything you pack weighs something and takes up space, and you're the one who's going to be dealing with this suitcase.

2 Buy small clear containers and bottles for your cosmetics, and take the minimum possible. You do not need to take full-sized anything, and some of these beauty items can be very heavy.

3 Wear your heaviest shoes on the plane, and pack as few pairs as possible. They add a lot of weight and can shift around during travel, making your suitcase unwieldy.

4 Don't pack your suitcase on the floor. Place the suitcase on your bed or, even better, on a higher, firm surface, such as a dining room table, so you don't have to lean over with every item you plan to pack. If you do use the bed, sit down next to the suitcase when packing.

5 Make sure the weight is distributed evenly inside the suitcase so it won't topple over. Reaching over to grab a falling suitcase is a good way to stress your lower back!

Carrying Your Luggage

Refer to the tips in the section Loading and Unloading the Trunk on pp. 161–162, as those apply to luggage as well.

1 Use luggage that is lightweight but sturdy. It should roll on thick and sturdy wheels and have a long handle that is comfortable to pull for your height. If not, you can buy extenders for the handle (like those for lawn mowers) to make it easy to pull.

2 Luggage with wheels is a lifesaver, and if you can, find a suitcase that you can push instead of pull, which puts even less strain on your back. If you can only pull your rolling suitcase, be sure you switch your hands when pulling, and keep your palms facedown to lessen the stress on your shoulders. Keep your abdominals contracted, and don't forget to breathe normally. This is especially important when you're pulling a suitcase, as twisting your body without thinking about it, especially when you're pulling a rolling object, can cause pain. Contracted abdominals will make this much less of a worry.

❸ If you must carry your luggage, keep it close to your body. Switch sides frequently, even if you're carrying only one bag, and try to keep the weight evenly distributed.

❹ Remember—just because your suitcase has wheels doesn't mean there will be no strain on your back. Go easy, never yank and give yourself extra time so you don't have to rush. When hurrying to get through security or to your gate, you'll likely forget to think about what you're doing.

How to Put Luggage in or Remove It from the Overhead Bin

Mass transit is not kind to anyone who needs to hoist their bags up. One wrong move and you can hurt your lower back, especially if you are short and need to strain to get the bags up in the air and onto a shelf or in a bin.

❶ When you're about to hoist the suitcase up into the bin, contract your abdominals and keep breathing normally.

❷ Turn to face the overhead bin, bring your suitcase up to chest height, then place it on the top of the aisle seat, where the headrest is (or on the seat if the suitcase is too big, so you can readjust it, if need be, before bringing it back up to chest height). Go up on your toes and slide the suitcase into the bin.

❸ If someone is already sitting in the aisle seat and you can't do step 2, make sure that you contract your abdominals before bringing the suitcase up to chest height, going up on your toes and placing it in the bin.

❹ To remove your suitcase, contract your abdominals, go up on your toes, slowly reach for the suitcase, pull it gently toward your chest and then adjust accordingly. Never yank or pull, and ignore the rumblings of passengers in line behind you if you need to take your time to do this carefully and properly! If you are short or in pain, ask for help.

How to Remove Luggage from the Conveyor Belt

Like loading or unloading the car trunk, this maneuver often causes lower back pain, because it involves leaning over and pulling up, in this case from a moving surface in a crowd of people. It's hard to have Back Mindfulness after a long and tiring flight, when you just want to get your suitcases and get out of the airport, but it's extremely important to remember to keep your abdominal muscles contracted, to breathe normally and to never yank or pull your suitcases with your legs straight.

1 If you can get a cart, do so. Carts take the edge off all the potentially stressful hauling, so always try to use one.

2 Make sure you are as close to the conveyor belt as possible. Stand away from others so you have room to maneuver properly.

3 Contract your abdominals, bend your knees slightly and go into a squat position. Bring your suitcase up as close to your body as you can, and slowly pivot your body away from the belt. You can also try a straddle position, which is a squat with your feet wider than shoulder-width apart and your toes pointed out, so you can get as close to the conveyor belt as possible. Cara uses this maneuver whenever she flies, and by now she is used to some of the peculiar looks thrown her way, but protecting your back is a lot more important than the opinion of strangers you'll never see again!

4 Once you have lifted your suitcase off the belt, bring it up to your waist before gently placing it on the floor. Breathe normally, and then contract your abdominals and bend your knees before lifting the luggage onto the cart. This might seem like a lot of different moves, but repositioning your body helps when you need to lift heavy bags.

Use a Backpack as a Carry-on

Many companies make lightweight yet durable backpacks. Using one might not be the most stylish thing in the world, but a backpack with wide straps, worn high up on your back, is much less stressful for your lower back than carrying an overloaded handbag and carry-on bag. Place the heaviest items closest to your back so they don't pull you backward. When taking the backpack off, ease it down gently so you don't twist your back.

Women who prefer to carry a handbag and a carry-on should switch sides every few minutes to relieve stress on their shoulders.

TOP TIPS FOR MANAGING BACK PAIN ON AN AIRPLANE

If you're of a certain age, you remember the glory days when commercial flying was a glamorous adventure, without endless security lines, cramped seating, and surly and exhausted fellow travelers trying to cram their too-large carry-ons into the overhead bins to avoid checked-luggage fees. Those days, unfortunately, are long gone, and flying can be a very stressful experience, no matter how much you're looking forward to a vacation or a visit to your family. Factor in lower back pain, and your trip can become hellacious, especially for frequent business fliers, who must endure the airports and the airplanes with little downtime for much-needed recovery.

As ever, a little Back Mindfulness goes a very long way toward relieving the misery!

Back-Friendly Flying Tips

❶ Try to fly in comfortable clothes. This means women should leave the tight jeans and the high heels at home, and men should wear well-tailored clothes that are not too tight around the waist.

If possible, loosen your belt so it's not constricting, or remove it altogether.

❷ Be sure to remove everything from your back pockets before you sit down.

❸ Try to reserve an aisle, bulkhead or exit row seat, as you'll have more legroom.

❹ If you're not in pain and if there's time before you board, walk around the airport as much as possible, and then do some of the standing stretches if you have adequate space (the Quadriceps Standing Stretch, the Hip Flexors Stretch and the Total Back Stretch). It can be difficult to find the space you need for these stretches on an airplane.

❺ Once on the airplane, get up as much as possible and walk up and down the aisles.

❻ While waiting to get off the airplane, if you're not in an aisle seat, remain seated until you can get up and stand straight. Otherwise, you will have to stand in a crouched position, which is terrible for your lower back. It's much better to wait a few minutes than to add more stress to what has already been a long journey.

❼ If you are having an episode of lower back pain yet you must fly, get a note from your physician stating that you are in pain and ask for additional help at the airport. This is not the time to be shy! Airlines have wheelchairs and motorized carts specifically for passengers who need them. Some airports are enormous, with very long distances between gates, which necessitates a lot of walking (and your airplane always seems to be at the gate farthest from security when your back is hurting, doesn't it!). You can be met at check-in or security, wheeled to the gate, and given extra time to get on the airplane. You might even get preferential seating. Call your airline prior to leaving for information and advice.

How to Get into an Airplane Seat

❶ You might have to squeeze in if you don't have an aisle seat, which usually involves hunching over. When booking flights, always try to get an aisle seat. Be sure to contract your abdominals and slightly bend your legs as you move from the aisle to your seat.

2 To sit down, hold onto the headrest of the seat in front of your own, contract your abdominals, bend your knees, and stick your buttocks out so that your hips move back and your buttocks touch the back of the seat.

3 When in your seat, lean forward slightly and place a pillow, if there is one, in a comfortable spot at your back for additional lumbar support, which, as you already know, can relieve stress on your lower back. If you can get more than one pillow, place the other one behind your head. Many travelers like to use lightweight blow-up neck pillows, as they help relieve strain on your neck and shoulders. If there's no pillow, you can use a sweatshirt, blanket, sweater or towel instead.

4 Place something sturdy under your feet for support. If you're not allowed to place anything on the floor, slip your feet out of your shoes and rest them on top of the shoes themselves for slight elevation. Or remove the magazines from the pouch of the seat in front of you and rest your feet on them. Or try taking your shoes off and resting your feet or your toes on the top of the magazine pouch, if it is sturdy enough.

BACK-SAVING ROUTINE FOR AIRPLANE TRAVEL

As airplane travel can force you to remain seated in back-stressing positions in a confined space over what can be a long period of time, you need to apply Back Mindfulness and make any necessary adjustments to ensure that you are as comfortable as possible and to reduce and/or eliminate pain.

If you can't do all the stretches on the airplane, at the very least, reposition your spine. Contract your abdominals and roll your pelvis forward, then backward, until you find the sweet spot where it feels comfortable for you. You may have to readjust your position like this throughout the flight, but doing so could save you time spent nursing your back, leaving you free to enjoy your final destination once you have landed.

Remember to get up and move around at least every thirty minutes, and do the following stretches and movements whenever you feel tight. If you're on a very long flight, you might want to do the entire sequence a few times.

1. Abdominal Contraction

1 Sit with your feet flat on the floor or go up on your toes, with your back touching the back of the seat and your hands on your belly.

2 Inhale, and then, on the exhale, contract your abdominals. Hold the contraction for five to ten seconds, and then release.

3 Do this ten times. You can do more if you like—just be sure not to hold your breath.

2. Pelvic Tilt

1 Sit tall on a chair with your feet flat on the floor or go up on your toes, with your back touching the back of the seat and your hands on your belly. Relax and make sure you are breathing normally.

2 Inhale, and then, on the exhale, contract your abdominals and tilt your pelvis back.

3 Hold the contraction and the position for three to five seconds, and then release slowly.

4 Do this ten times.

3. Shoulder Shrug

1 Sit with your feet flat on the floor or go up on your toes, with your back touching the back of the seat and your arms by your sides.

2 Inhale, and then, on the exhale, contract your abdominals.

3 Slowly raise your shoulders up toward your ears, hold for a few seconds, and then slowly lower them. It should take three seconds to go up and three seconds to go down.

4 Do this five to ten times.

For the next two exercises, pick whichever one you feel comfortable doing.

4a. Seated Twist

1 Sit tall with your feet flat on the floor, hip-width apart, your back touching the back of the seat, and your arms at your sides.

2 Inhale, and then, on the exhale, contract your abdominals.

3 Cross your left leg over your right leg, and then place both arms over to your left side and slowly twist at your waist so you can look over at your right shoulder.

4 Hold this position for ten seconds, and then switch to your left side.

5 Do this two times.

6 If this stretch bothers your neck, cross your left leg over your right knee and, with your right hand, grab the armrest on your left. Hold this position for ten seconds, and then switch sides. This variation does not involve your neck.

4b. Side Stretch

Do this only if there's room overhead.

1 Sit with your feet flat on the floor, your back touching the back of the seat.

2 Inhale, and then, on the exhale, contract your abdominals.

3 Hold on to the left side of your seat with your left hand, and then slowly bring your right arm over your head.

4 Hold this position for ten seconds, and then switch to your left side.

5 Do this two times.

5. Piriformis Stretch

Do this only if armrests are not in the way.

1 Sit tall with your feet flat on the floor.

2 Inhale, and then, on the exhale, contract your abdominals.

3 Cross your right leg over your left leg so that your right ankle is resting on your left thigh.

4 Place your right hand on your right knee and your left hand on your right ankle. Bring your upper body down toward your right leg. Stop leaning down as soon as you feel the stretch in the right piriformis muscle, located on the side of your right hip and buttock. Do not round your back.

5 Hold this position for fifteen seconds, and then switch sides, crossing your left leg over your right leg.

6. Headrest Reach

1 Sit with your feet flat on the floor, and then raise your heels and go up on your toes, keeping them pointed down.

2 Inhale, and then, on the exhale, contract your abdominals and do a Pelvic Tilt.

3 Stretch your hands toward the headrest in front of you, and hold this position for five seconds. Return to the starting position.

4 If you can't stretch your arms out in front of you, then raise them straight up, follow the first two steps and hold for five seconds.

CHAPTER 8

MANAGING YOUR BACK PAIN AND YOUR FAMILY

WITH ALL THE DEMANDS of modern life, it's hard enough to be a parent on a good day. It's even harder on a bad day, when your back is aching so much, you can't even pick up your toddler for a goodnight kiss. This chapter will show you how to manage back pain when you are pregnant and when you need to lift, push or carry children; and how to incorporate Back Mindfulness whenever you shop or go out.

PREGNANCY AND LOWER BACK PAIN

Pregnancy is a tremendous joy—but that happiness can be tempered by tremendous suffering if the pregnancy triggers an episode of lower back pain or makes existing pain worse. A strong core is very important to our back health and overall health, and this is especially true for pregnant women. Many women come to my office with marked discomfort in their second or third trimester, usually because at that point the fetus is growing rapidly and its weight puts additional stress on a woman's back. This pain can be difficult to treat as X-rays are not recommended during pregnancy (except for emergencies), and neither are many prescription medications for pain. In addition, many exercises cannot safely be done at various points during a pregnancy, so you must always seek expert advice from your obstetrician about activities you can and cannot do.

What Pregnancy Does to Your Lower Back

Many changes happen to a woman's body as her pregnancy progresses:

- Your center of gravity shifts forward due to the additional weight of the fetus in your abdomen. As a result, many women lean back as a counterbalance, and this makes it more difficult to maintain a neutral spine position.

- Your abdominal muscles stretch to accommodate the growing fetus, and this places additional stress on your back muscles, so if these are already weak, they will have more strain put upon them. As you know, when additional stressors are placed on your core, the erector muscles of your back can become hard and tight, causing intense pain.

- As your uterus expands, it can put more pressure on your spine, therefore increasing the chances of sciatica.

- A hormone called relaxin is released to loosen the ligaments in parts of your body, primarily those attached to the weight-bearing joints in your pelvis, to facilitate the movement of the fetus as it passes through the pelvis during delivery. This flexibility is needed during labor, but it's one of the reasons why any exercise during pregnancy might need to be modified and why you need expert advice from your obstetrician about what activities are safe.

- Sleeping on your back with additional weight centered in your abdomen places additional stress on your back muscles, which must support it.

Top Tips to Help Your Lower Back During Pregnancy

Ideally, if you stretch every day and your core is strong before you become pregnant, your core will respond better to the additional stress load placed upon it during pregnancy. This flexibility and strength will also aid you during delivery, as your ability to physically deliver your child stems from your core. For those with a normal delivery, it should be much easier to push, and your muscle recovery should be swifter.

- Do the seven stretches and the core routine per your obstetrician's advice. Any moves that involve your core muscles during pregnancy should be discussed prior to starting any stretching or exercise routine, even if you are already an experienced exerciser or athlete.

- Back Mindfulness is needed now more than ever, especially during your third trimester—but, of course, you have a lot on your mind! But do your best to move in a way that will keep your lower back as protected as possible.

- Be sure to lift properly. Never bend over at a ninety-degree angle with straight legs, as this is bad for your lower back on a good day, and is particularly stressful with additional fetus weight in your abdomen.

- Take a lot of breaks when doing regular household chores. Elevate your feet if they get swollen.

- Make sure that your chair and workstation are as ergonomically designed as possible. This is especially important if you're working at a desk during your pregnancy. Get up and move around frequently. For more tips, see pp. 141–143 in Chapter 6.

- Use a lumbar cushion or a firm pillow while sitting, and try to maintain your neutral spine position.

- Do Kegel exercises, as these will strengthen the muscles of your pelvic floor.

- Be aware of your sleeping position. If you are a back sleeper, you can relieve some of the pressure by placing pillows under your knees, or between your knees, if you prefer to sleep on your side. Be sure to speak to your obstetrician about back sleeping, as it might not be advisable after your first trimester. Or even better, make a nest of pillows as described in the sidebar on p. 178.

Lifting during Pregnancy

1. Get as close as possible to the object before you lift it. Place your feet shoulder-width apart, and make sure you have a firm footing.

2. Contract your abdominals and keep them contracted the entire time, while breathing normally.

3. Slowly bend your knees and squat down. Try to get the object between your legs when possible so you don't have too far to reach.

4. Slowly lift the object up. Do not drop your head; keep your eyes focused forward. Do your best not to make any jerking movements when you're lifting. Bring the object up to chest height, and then slowly rise up.

5. Or you can kneel down on one leg, if this doesn't bother your knee, and bring the object as close to your body as possible. Bring the object up to chest height, and, then slowly rise up.

To place an object down, reverse the steps.

Use a Nest of Pillows to Support Your Back in Bed

As you read on p.128 in Chapter 5, a nest of pillows can make sleeping much more comfortable.

Back Sleepers
Place one or two pillows under your knees and neck, and one or two under each arm. Make sure your neck is not strained. You might need to experiment with different pillows to find the perfect balance.

Side Sleepers
Sleeping on your side, particularly in a fetal position, is advised after your first trimester, rather than sleeping on your back, but if this bothers your knees, make sure to place a pillow between your legs, as this

will cushion the weight of your top leg so it won't feel so heavy on top of your bottom leg. Place one pillow between your knees, one or two pillows on your right side, one or two pillows on your left side (this cradles you), and one or two pillows (one is preferable) under your head, whichever is most comfortable and does not put any strain on your neck and back. Experiment with pillows of different sizes and densities to create the best nest for your back.

BEFORE YOU START YOUR STRETCHES AND CORE ROUTINE

1 Empty your bladder before doing the routines.

2 Warm up for five to ten minutes before starting.

3 Stay hydrated.

4 Wear a good supportive bra and nonrestrictive clothing.

5 Stop if you feel any discomfort, pain or anything unusual.

7 STRETCHES FOR PREGNANCY

Before you start, remember to use caution. *Always* check with your obstetrician *before* doing any stretches or core exercises, or any form of physical activity. This is especially important whenever you do any activities that involve abdominal contractions. During pregnancy, you are stretching and exercising for one—but the risk is always for two.

Once you have been given the go-ahead by your obstetrician, try to do these stretches once a day.

1. Chest Opener

1 Stand facing a sturdy pole, the edge of a doorway or a wall, and grab hold of it with your right hand.

2 Contract your abdominals, and then slowly pivot your foot and rotate your body to your left, away from the pole, doorway or wall (which will now be behind you). You should feel the stretch in your chest, just above your right breast.

3 Hold the stretch for fifteen seconds, and then switch to your left side. Remember to keep breathing evenly.

2. Shoulder Shrug

1 Sit with your feet flat on the floor or up on your toes, or you can elevate your feet with a stool, if this makes you feel more comfortable. Your back should touch the back of the chair, and your arms should be by your sides.

2 Inhale, and then, on the exhale, contract your abdominals.

3 Slowly raise your shoulders up toward your ears, hold for a few seconds, and then slowly lower them. It should take three seconds to go up and three seconds to go down.

4 Do this ten times.

3. Standing Hamstring Stretch

1 Stand upright, facing a chair, step or stool.

2 Inhale, and then, on the exhale, pull your belly in and place your right heel on the chair seat, step or stool.

3 Place your right hand on your right leg and your left hand on your left leg. If you need more support, place the chair or stool near a wall or sturdy furniture.

4 Slightly bend your left knee, and slowly lower your upper body down toward your right leg. Hold the stretch for fifteen to thirty seconds.

5 Slowly raise your upper body until you are upright, and remove your right foot from the chair, step or stool. Repeat with your left leg.

6 Do this two times.

4. Seated Piriformis Stretch

1 Sit tall on a chair with your feet flat on the floor, hip-width apart, your back touching the back of the chair.

2 Inhale, and then, on the exhale, contract your abdominals and cross your right leg over your left leg so that your right ankle is resting on your left thigh.

3 Place your right hand on your right ankle and your left hand on your right knee. Slowly lower your upper body, pressing on your right leg. Stop lowering yourself as soon as you feel the stretch in the right piriformis muscle, located on the right side of your hip and buttock. Do not round your back.

④ Hold this position for fifteen seconds, and then switch, crossing your left leg over your right leg.

For the next four exercises, pick whichever one you feel comfortable doing.

5a. Hip Flexors Stretch

❶ Place a pillow on the floor and kneel down, placing your left knee on top of the pillow. (If you are on a carpet or mat, you can do this without a pillow, if you prefer.)

❷ Step forward with your right knee, while keeping your left knee on the floor. If you're worried about your balance, either rest both hands on a sturdy chair placed at your side or place your hands on the floor, on either side of your front leg.

❸ Slide your left leg behind you until you feel the stretch in the front of your left hip. Make sure your right knee does not go beyond your foot (to protect your knee joint).

④ Hold this position for thirty seconds.

❺ Switch sides and repeat.

5b. Hip Flexor One Cheek Chair Stretch – Variation 2

❶ Stand with a sturdy chair on your right side, and then place only your right buttock on the seat. Keep your right leg bent in front of you.

❷ Slide your left leg behind you to get a comfortable stretch in the front of your left hip.

3 Hold this position for thirty seconds.

4 Switch sides and repeat.

6. Quadriceps Standing Stretch

1 Stand next to a sturdy piece of furniture, and hold on to it for balance with your left hand.

2 Grasp your right foot (or ankle, if that's easier) with your right hand, and gently pull your leg back and up, with your toes pointing toward your head. Make sure your knee remains straight and close to your left leg. It should not move out toward your right side.

3 Hold this position for thirty seconds.

4 Switch to your left leg and repeat.

5 Do this two times.

7. Total Back Stretch

1 Stand next to a sturdy chair, knees bent. Slowly pull in your belly, and then grasp the chair with both hands, keeping your arms straight. Keep your head level with your shoulders.

2 Hold this position for ten seconds.

3 Stand up straight, place your right hand on your waist and your left arm up over your head, and then bend to the right. You can use the chair for support if you need to.

4 Hold this position for ten seconds, and then switch sides.

TAKING CARE OF YOUR CHILDREN

Now that your pregnancy is over and you have already shed some of the baby weight, which may have been causing lower back pain, along with the love and happiness can come a whole new set of fears. When it comes to your back, how do you hold the baby properly? How do you lift up or put down a baby when your back hurts? How can you make sure you never drop the baby?

You can make it easier and more reassuring for yourself if you have good upper-body strength prior to giving birth. Always speak to your obstetrician first, and if you're given the go-head, start doing simple weight-lifting exercises to strengthen your arms, shoulders, legs and upper back while you are pregnant, in addition to doing the stretches in this chapter. It is not advisable to do strength training by yourself during pregnancy if you have no experience with it. Be sure to work with a qualified trainer to make sure you are doing these exercises properly, especially as your center of gravity shifts with your expanding belly.

How to Lift the Baby out of the Crib

Even if your back is hurting, you can still lift and nurture your baby—as long as you do it properly. Since new cribs are no longer allowed to have a drop-down side due to safety concerns over entrapment, anyone suffering from back pain needs to have a safe and effective means of leaning over to pick up a baby in a crib or anywhere else.

As you read in the Lift It Right section on pp. 62–63 in Chapter 2, the worst lifting technique for your lower back is to bend forward with your legs straight and then lift with your spine in a flexed position. This puts you at a ninety-degree angle. All the force of the lift is vectored right to your lower back.

Instead, you can disperse the weight of the baby you're lifting throughout all the muscles of your body by following these three steps.

❶ Get as close to the crib as possible. If it's an older crib and you can lower the side, do so now.

❷ Instead of leaning over with your knees straight, bend them slightly and contract your abdominals.

❸ Pick up the baby slowly, and then bring him or her as close to your chest as possible. Only then should you straighten your knees.

Holding and Lifting Infants, Toddlers and Older Children

❶ Be sure to bend with your knees, not your waist, and then squat down to pick the child up from a position as close to the child as possible. Contract your abdominals, and bring the child as close to your body, at chest height, as possible.

❷ Hold your child so he or she is centered on your body, instead of on one hip. But if you do not feel comfortable doing this and opt for your hip, then make sure you switch hips every so often.

❸ A worthwhile investment is a rocking chair or a gliding rocker. Mothers through the ages have soothed their children and themselves by rocking, as a rocking motion modulates the central nervous system, which then relaxes your neuromuscular system. Try a few rockers when you're in a baby store, and buy one that is the most comfortable for your body. Most of them are firm and have good lumbar support. Be sure to prop your feet up on a stool when you're sitting on a rocker.

Infant Carriers, Slings, Strollers, Diaper Bags and Car Seats

Infant Carriers

Infant carriers do a great job of protecting your newborn, but are not easy on your back when carried. They are unavoidable, as many hospitals will not let you leave without a sturdy carrier that snaps into a car seat. Most people use one arm to hold this carrier, and the awkward, bulky shape pulls your shoulder out of alignment and twists your back. As hard as it may be, try to have someone else hold this carrier with its precious cargo whenever possible.

If you do have to lift this carrier up, use both hands. Keep your abdominals contracted, and carry it close to your body. Try to carry using both hands, but if that is uncomfortable, use one hand, but switch to the other side every few minutes. Keep your abdominals contracted the entire time. Don't twist with your legs straight; keep them slightly bent.

If you are out and have been carrying the carrier for a while and are aching, try to do as much stretching as you can, but if you're pressed for time and space, these two stretches should loosen you up a bit until you get home to do the 7 Pregnancy Stretches.

First, put the baby carrier down safely next to you on a flat surface.

1. Chest Opener

❶ Stand facing a sturdy pole, the edge of a doorway or a wall, and grab hold of it with your right hand.

❷ Contract your abdominals, and then slowly pivot your foot and rotate your body to your left, away from the pole, doorway or wall (which will now be behind you). You should feel the stretch in your chest, just above your right breast.

❸ Hold the stretch for fifteen seconds, and then switch to your left side. Remember to keep breathing evenly.

2. Shoulder Pull

❶ Stand with your feet hip-width apart, and then contract your abdominals.

❷ Bring your right arm across your body to your left side, hold your right elbow with your left hand and pull in toward your body.

❸ Hold the stretch for five seconds, and then switch to your left arm. You will feel this in the front of your shoulder.

Slings

If you ever have episodes of back pain before your baby is born, and you're worried about carrying your baby, try going to a baby store while you are still pregnant. Ask for advice about the most ergonomic baby slings. Try on different slings and put in a few large cans of formula, as that will approximate the weight of a baby so you can get an idea of how the sling feels on your body.

Many women like the front-carrying slings, such as the BabyBjörn, and have no problems with them causing any back pain. Others prefer a hip sling, as it distributes the baby's weight differently; still others prefer a more rigid backpack-type carrier that rides high on the back (which is better for older babies and toddlers). You can check recommendations online.

Strollers

When buying a stroller, look for one that is very easy to collapse, ideally with one hand. Struggling to fold and hoist a stroller, especially when holding a baby with one arm, can be very stressful for anyone with back pain. It is also crucial to check the height of the handles. If the handles seem too low, improvise by putting something over the handles to elevate your hands, such as a piece of foam that you can wrap around the handles. Handles vary considerably, and you want to make sure the stroller can be pushed easily, without you needing to reach up (if you're short) or slouch over (if you're tall). The last thing you want to do is strain your back merely by going out for a walk with your baby in the stroller!

When pushing the stroller, be conscious of your posture. Use Back Mindfulness, and don't hunch over the handles. Be sure to check with your obstetrician first about when it is safe to push a stroller after delivery, and once you are given the go-ahead, which is often after at least six to eight weeks, try to engage your abdominals as you walk—this will not only strengthen your muscles but will also help tone areas that were stretched during pregnancy.

Diaper Bags

There are countless varieties of diaper bags, but we recommend you choose function over fashion in order to keep your back strong and safe. Loading in all the stuff your baby seems to need can quickly make these bags a real strain on your shoulders and back. Try to pare down to essentials only.

If you use a shoulder diaper bag, be sure to alternate sides every few minutes. This is such a simple and easy step that few women remember to do (ditto with overloaded handbags!), but it can make a big difference.

You might also want to try using a backpack-type diaper bag, as this will keep the weight evenly distributed. It won't work if you have the baby in a sling, but it can be helpful if you're pushing a stroller. If so, try to keep the heavy items in the bottom of the stroller.

Car Seats

Like getting in and out of bed or on and off the toilet, car seats are something you have to deal with whether your back hurts or not. Unfortunately, there is no getting around the fact that car seats and back pain do not mix! Placing the baby in the seat and managing the buckles means you have to lean over, lean down and twist, but your baby's safety is paramount, so you don't have a choice.

❶ If possible, open the car door before you take the baby out of the carrier, stroller or sling.

When you're holding the baby, keep him or her as close to your body as possible, as this will reduce the stress on your lower back.

❷ Contract your abdominals. Instead of leaning in with the baby and twisting to place him or her in the seat, turn with your back to the front seat and actually step into the backseat with one foot (or both feet, if you have the space) so that you are facing the car seat.

❸ Contract your abdominals and keep breathing. Then brace your back against the front seat, and you will have that support keeping you steady as you lean forward slightly to place the baby in the car seat.

❹ Repeat when taking the baby out of the car seat.

OUTSIDE ACTIVITIES

For many people, shopping is a relaxing and enjoyable way to spend time and buy things they need and want. For others, it is a necessary annoyance that's done as quickly as possible. Yet for all shoppers, Back Mindfulness is a must. When you're busy looking at merchandise or trying things on, you are probably not thinking about your back—but all the bending, reaching and twisting movement you are doing, especially when bending over to strap on some new shoes, can set your back on fire.

Shopping

If you're a typical female shopper, this is what you likely do: you carry an overloaded handbag on one shoulder and do not switch sides; when looking for items to try on, you rummage through the rack for your size or favored styles; and when you finally find what you like, that usually means using one hand to push the other clothes out of the way, bending over a table to pick items up, or reaching overhead to pull items down. Then, if you're pressed for time, as most people usually are, you proceed to pile as many articles of clothing in your arms as you can carry, most likely on one side of your body, because you need a free hand to keep your handbag in place and to perhaps pick up other items. And you haven't even walked into the dressing room yet.

Once inside the dressing room, you start hanging your clothes up on a tiny hook, which means more bending, twisting and reaching, and even more of these movements when you put on and take off multiple garments in a short span of time. You might also have to bend down to take off your shoes. Remember to breathe and watch your back!

How to Try on Clothes

These tips should help prevent back pain while shopping:

1 Stretch before you leave the house.

2 Take only the most lightweight essentials in a small, equally light-weight handbag. Sling it over one shoulder and across your body, if possible, as this will keep the weight off your shoulders and will free up both hands. If not, be sure to switch sides often.

3 Wear comfortable clothes and shoes that are easy to take on and off. You might be doing a lot of walking, and you certainly don't want to stride across the department store in high heels, with your arms full of heavy clothing.

4 Take your time rummaging through the racks.

5 When doing any kind of bending, twisting or reaching, remember to contract your abdominal muscles. Breathe normally.

6 Also remember to keep your knees slightly bent and to squat down slowly when picking up something on a low table. Never bend to pick something up with straight legs! If you need to reach up, go up on your toes, rather than stretching your arms, with your feet flat on the floor. Do not twist or turn while reaching.

7 Ask for help. This can be difficult when salespeople seem to evaporate as soon as you arrive, but you can try asking someone at a register to watch some of your garments so you don't have to carry a heavy pile. If you do see a salesperson, ask for assistance putting the garments in the dressing room.

8 Look for a dressing room with a three-way mirror, which is not always the most flattering but prevents you from having to twist to look at your back.

9 If there is a chair in the dressing room, use that to drape the clothes on so you don't have to hang them up; you'll do a lot less reaching. If there is enough space, you can even use this chair to brace yourself when you do the stretches in the sidebar on p. 191. You will already be warmed up!

10 Instead of bending over to try on clothes, lean against the door or any of the walls when putting on clothes, while contracting your abdominals.

⑪ As soon as your shopping bags start to accumulate, make a trip back to your car. (Remember to follow the tips about placing items in the trunk on pp. 161–162 in Chapter 7.) You'll lessen the stress on your back from having to carry a lot of bags plus reap the aerobic rewards of the extra walking.

⑫ Stretch when you get home, or at least before bed.

Stretches for Shopping

When you do these stretches, you should feel some relief from the tightness shopping can bring on. If you start to get that familiar feeling of strain in your lower back, and you have time for only one stretch, do #3, the Pelvic Release.

1. Shoulder Shrug — See p. 147

When shopping, do this only two to three times. If you can't find a chair, stand with your feet hip-width apart and your arms down by your sides before starting the stretch.

2. Standing Side Stretch

❶ Stand with your feet hip-width apart, and then place your left hand on your left hip and bend over to the left with your right arm overhead.

❷ Hold this position for three to five seconds, and then switch to your right side.

❸ Do this two or three times.

---

3. Standing Pelvic Release on the Wall

❶ Stand with your back against a wall, legs slightly bent. Your feet should be shoulder-width apart, about one foot from the wall.

❷ Contract your abdominals and roll your pelvis backward—this will press your lower back into the wall. Hold this position for three to five seconds.

❸ Do this two or three times.

How to Try on Shoes

Shoe shopping can be particularly stressful for your back. Many women try a new shoe on one foot while still wearing their old shoe on the other, which automatically puts them out of alignment, and then they walk around with mismatched shoes, which makes things worse. Keep in mind the seating in shoe shops is usually at a peculiar height, which means you have to lean forward to deal with the box and packaging and to adjust the new shoes, and that you'll be thinking about the shoes, and not your back, as you lean over and then stand up to admire them or check the fit. If the heels are high, this will automatically cause your pelvis to tip forward, which is guaranteed to place additional stress on your back.

Follow these tips for pain-free shoe shopping:

❶ As tempting as it may be, don't try on the display shoe. Try on only your size.

❷ Stand for as long as you can in the shoes. Sit only when you are actually trying the shoes on, even if you're tired, unless standing bothers your back. Keep your bag off your shoulder when trying anything on.

❸ Put the shoe boxes on the chair next to you, not on the floor.

④ If you can't use the chair next to you, contract your abdominals, place your feet on tiptoes and reach down to get the box. Open the box when it's on your lap, *not* on the floor.

⑤ Put the box down and keep the shoes in your lap. Try each one on by bringing your leg up, not bending down to the floor.

⑥ When you're ready to stand up and walk around in the new shoes, contract your abdominals, grab the armrests (if possible) for support, lean forward slightly, and push yourself up, using your hands and legs.

⑦ After walking around, sit back down and bring one knee up at a time to remove the shoes. Do not bend down to take them off.

⑧ If your back is starting to bother you, try doing a Quadriceps Standing Stretch, a Seated Twist and a Piriformis Stretch. They're quick and easy and might just allow you to continue with your shopping.

⑨ If you're shopping for shoes as well as for other items, do the shoe shopping first, as it causes the most stress on your back. As with clothes shopping, if you have several bags of shoes, take them to your car and then return to the store! And don't forget how to carry the bags properly (see pp. 189–191).

Attack of the Killer High Heels

If you are a fan of the *Sex and the City* television series, you might remember the scene when Carrie is allowed into the secret *Vogue* magazine clothes closet. When she sees the Manolo Blahnik shoes lined up on the shelves, she is stunned into ecstasy. I know how women, like Carrie, can obsess about their shoes: they often discuss which pairs they love so much that they keep wearing them even though they exacerbate their back pain. As a spine surgeon, however, I have to say that choosing style over pain is not something I would ever recommend, especially as there are countless shoe styles that are both comfortable and great looking.

Which shoes are the best for me? is a question to ask your back doctor, as well as your podiatrist, but suffice it to say that high heels do no woman's body any good. They may make your legs look longer and sexier, but they are hell for your feet, ankles, knees and back. And very flat shoes without any arch support, as is commonly found in ballerina-style flats, can also be bad for your feet and lower back.

The best kind of shoe to wear—and especially when you have back pain—is one that has a well-supported arch and heel. So look for shoes that have good, supportive arches, that fit well, that have adequate cushioning and that have a low heel or a low wedge heel. You don't want any shoe with either a high heel or a flat or very low heel, and thus no arch support at all, although if your feet have naturally high arches, this might bother you less.

Going to the Movies or the Theater

If you have great seats at the theater that rarely means that the seats themselves are great. In fact, theater and movie seats are often a backache waiting to happen, as they have been designed to maximize space for theater owners, not for patrons. Remember, even if it's during a very pleasurable activity—like a theatrical production you've been looking forward to seeing for a long time—you're still sitting!

So what can you do to make your seats more ergonomic when you have no control over the seating? Bringing your own lumbar support pillow or cushion may help. In a movie theater or a drama theater, try to get an aisle seat, so you can stretch out your legs a bit. You can also try standing in the back of the theater (some Broadway theaters actually sell highly discounted standing-room tickets), and try walking a bit in the back while viewing a movie.

If you're stuck in your seat, contract your abdominals as often as you can. (There's no limit to how often you can do this!) Try to fidget discreetly as much as possible, or do a Seated Pelvic Tilt to release the tension. If there's no one in the seat in front of you, try resting your feet on the armrests, even if only for a few minutes. If you must cross your legs, switch legs every few minutes.

Walking Your Dog

For many people, having a dog is great for their health if they go out for regular walks. These walks are an excellent way to warm yourself up before doing your stretches and core exercises.

But dog walking can be very taxing on your back, because you are walking with a moving object pulling you—and this delightful moving object might be prone to darting all over the place, because that's just what dogs do! It doesn't matter whether the dog is a toy poodle or a Great Dane—the randomness of the pulling and jerking is the issue. Of course, a big dog is more likely to pull you with great force, as opposed to a little dog, but you still need to be careful, no matter what its size. Here are a few tips:

- Make sure your dog is obedience trained, as this makes for a much calmer and controllable dog when you go outside.

- Use a training leash that goes over the dog's snout rather than on his body or neck, as this gives you far more control over the dog and he will not be able to pull you easily.

- Switch sides so that you are not always holding the leash with your dominant hand.

- When you have to pick up the poop, remember to contract your abdominals and squat down slowly. Never bend forward with your legs straight. Or get a pooper-scooper that does the bending for you.

CHAPTER 9

MANAGING YOUR BACK PAIN AND EXERCISE/SPORTS

SPORTS ARE GREAT FUN and wonderful activities that keep our cardiovascular system functioning well and our muscles and bones strong and supple. But due to the many kinds of motions needed to play sports, athletes and those who work out have a greater risk of sustaining a lower back injury. With sports such as skiing, basketball, football, dance, ice-skating, soccer, running, golf and tennis, the spine endures a significant amount of stress and absorption of pressure, twisting, turning and even bodily impact during play.

An estimated 5 to 10 percent of athletic injuries involve the lower lumbar spine area, and most are simple strains. They're usually caused by a specific event or trauma, like overreaching for a backhand volley on the tennis court or getting tackled on the football field, though some are due to repetitive minor injuries that result in micro-trauma.

I can tell you categorically that most athletes deny or minimize their low back pain and do not seek medical help. This is especially true of professional athletes, and of course, it is understandable, as withdrawing from competition can mean a huge loss of income and a lower ranking.

Problems with sports and lower back pain often start in childhood. Nonspecific musculoskeletal pain is responsible for at least 50 percent of the cases of children and adolescents complaining of lower back pain. And a recent study of nearly 4,700 eighteen-year-old college students found that those who had been involved in sports since elementary school had a significantly higher rate of lower back pain than their less competitive peers. Overall 72 percent of students who had played sports since elementary school reported having had a bout of back pain, compared with 62 percent of those who had spent few years playing sports, and 50 percent of those who had never been involved in competitive sports.

Why is that? Because these kids haven't been training properly. They often don't warm up or cool down enough. They rarely, if ever, stretch. And certainly they rarely, if ever, have any training or competence in stretching (the only exception being dancers, gymnasts and figure skaters, whose daily classes incorporate stretching and muscle strengthening, which are needed for their sport).

In addition, athletes, no matter what their level, are take-charge and competitive by nature. They don't want to stop or even slow down. So they can sometimes forge ahead and live with the pain, until it's too late—and when it is, they'll almost always have to endure far more devastating and potentially chronic problems.

It's not been easy to convince athletes that most of their lower back pain can easily be treated with physical therapy and exercise, and that the seven stretches and core exercises will help them prevent subsequent damage, which could very well eventually lead to a permanent and career-ending injury. Often, they just don't want to listen, even when I tell them that research shows that improved conditioning absolutely reduces the incidence of not only lower back pain but also serious lumbar spine problems.

Professional athletes are not the only people who suffer from lower back pain. As you can imagine, it is also very common in the weekend warrior or sporadic exerciser, and in regular exercisers doing their best to stay healthy. Of course, it is always great to work out whenever possible, but you need to apply Back Mindfulness to any physical activity, including sports. It is especially important if you run and/or play racquet sports or, my passion, golf, which we'll explore in more detail in this chapter.

WHAT EXERCISE DOES TO YOUR LOWER BACK

On pp. 11–13 in Chapter 1, you read all about the motion segments of the lower lumbar spine—those cleverly designed bone-disc-bone facet complexes—so you know how they move physiologically, and how easy it can be to injure them. So let's see what athletic activity does to the motion segments and muscles of your lower back.

Open and Closed Chain Exercises

There are two types of exercise: open chain and closed chain. During an open chain exercise, such as running or tennis, your feet constantly leave the ground, and then when they make contact with the ground again, force is delivered to the lower lumbar spine, where the motion segments are. During closed chain exercises, such as riding a stationary bike or using a StairMaster, a stairstepper or an elliptical machine, your feet never leave the ground and there is no direct force delivered to the lower lumbar spine.

Due to the pounding nature of open-chain activity, there can be repetitive trauma to the disc spaces. In those who have weak muscles (especially in their core) or any form of degenerative disc problem, the chances increase that they will develop chronic lower back pain if they engage in open-chain exercise.

Running and Your Lower Back

Running is a very common and enjoyable sport for millions of people. Not only can it be stress relieving to go for a contemplative jog or a longer run before or after a tough day at work, but running provides an excellent cardiovascular workout, which is good for heart and lung health as well as weight loss. But because running is an open-chain exercise, it is very demanding on your lower lumbar spine. Your core must be strong for you to be able to balance yourself for an extended period of time when you run. Any muscle imbalances you have place stress on your spine when you run. In addition, running or jogging is an extension activity, meaning that your spine and pelvis are tilted backward, which puts significant pressure on the entire spine. Most runners or joggers run in this extended position, which puts repetitive compressive loads onto their spine's motion segments every time their feet leave and then hit the ground. Run like this for several miles at a time, multiple times a week, and eventually your back might start screaming in protest.

To avoid this, you want to run using perfect form. This means you should seek out your ideal neutral spine position, one in which your muscles all counterbalance each other so that you maintain a perfect alignment. If you hyperextend (your spine moves backward) or flex (your spine moves forward) due to fatigued muscles, this will cause even more stress to be placed on the lumbar spine, and not dispersed throughout your core muscles. Tired muscles also provide less support, as well as placing more pressure on the spine, which can also lead to damage to not only the discs themselves but also to the facet joints. When that happens, you are at increased risk for developing low back pain.

Lessening the Risk of Lower Back Pain When You Run

❶ You can effectively stabilize and support your spine, and overcome the trauma to it by the pounding nature of running activity, by increasing your core strength and stability. The stretches and core exercises in Chapters 2 and 3, as well as in this chapter, have been specifically designed to do this.

❷ Make sure that you have the best possible running shoes. They should fit properly, should not be worn down at the heel and should have good arch support, as this will help decrease the stresses to your lumbar spine.

❸ Always warm up properly.

❹ Try to keep your abdominals contracted when you run, as this will brace your spine better upon impact.

❺ Make sure you breathe properly.

❻ Know your course before you run. Unexpected hills, potholes, uneven pavement and wet surfaces can cause additional stress.

Racquet Sports and Your Lower Back

Tennis is a popular sport for all ages. The specific repetitive movements when serving and when hitting tennis balls are what make it so much fun, but this also means that tennis is notorious for causing lower back pain in recreational players as well as professionals.

More specifically, a tennis player goes through countless trunk rotations and twisting motions while performing forehand and backhand shots. While doing the normal routine of a forehand or a backhand shot, there is a change from extension to flexion, often while running and turning at the same time, and this creates a constant load on your spine's discs and facet-joint complexes. Not only that, but these shots are done with rapid start-and-stop motions, making tennis an open-chain exercise that places significant stress on the lumbar spine, especially as all these motions are absorbed by your lower back and pelvis. The back muscles must endure repeated sudden forward and lateral movements and the start/stop movements. It is almost impossible to think about Back Mindfulness in the less than split second it takes to go after a ball.

And then there's the overhead serve. This is done in a static position, but when throwing up the ball and then bringing your racquet down to hit it, it is necessary to hyperextend your lower back, which compresses the lumbar discs and the joints, which rely on the muscles around them to stabilize them. People who have weak core muscles will not be able to withstand this repetitive hyperextension. Eventually, they will develop lower back pain, and if it is not rectified, chronic lower back problems can result.

Lessening the Risk of Lower Back Pain When You Play Tennis

❶ As with running, you can effectively stabilize and support your spine when you play tennis, and overcome the trauma to it by the overhead and lateral motions of the sport, by increasing your core strength and stability. Do the stretches and core exercises in Chapters 2 and 3, as well as in this chapter.

❷ Make sure that you have the best possible tennis shoes for your feet. They should fit properly, should not be worn down at the heel and should have good arch support, as this will help decrease the stresses to your lumbar spine.

❸ Always warm up properly.

❹ Try to keep your abdominals contracted when you run as this will brace your spine better upon impact.

❺ Make sure you breathe properly.

6 Your racquet should be strung properly and should be the right size for your body/swing.

7 Never play on a wet court, as you will be prone to slipping, and this can be catastrophic for your back.

8 Watch how the professionals play. You should also seek professional training to ensure that you learn, or continue to play with, the best possible form. Doing so will not only improve your game but will also make injuries less likely.

9 Use proper lifting technique, as described in the Lift It Right section on pp. 62–63 in Chapter 2, when bending over to pick up the balls. If you are taking regular lessons, a metal ball holder that picks up the balls can be a real back saver.

Golf and Your Lower Back

Golf grows more and more popular every day. It's a wonderful sport that anyone, from kids to seniors, can enjoy—but it's also a sport that compromises the lower back like no other. It is widely believed that at least 80 percent of all amateurs play with lower back pain or get injured at some point in their playing days. This is especially true for older golfers. I've found that many of my patients are incredibly depressed about having to give up their cherished golf games because their back hurts too much during and after play. It has also been estimated that a whopping 90 percent of professional golfers suffer from lower back pain, and back pain is one of the leading disabilities on the PGA Tour.

In nearly all cases, golf-related lower back pain stems from improper postural alignment and muscle imbalance, either during play or from everyday life. The reason for all this pain is that the golf swing is a very traumatic motion for the entire body, but especially the lower back. There is significant torque involved in the proper mechanics of the swing. In order to hit a golf ball correctly and accurately, you must undertake an extremely complicated set of motions relying on many different muscle groups and then pivot through the lower back and the hips.

Golfers need to know about their "spine angle," which is the angle formed during a proper swing so you can hit the ball correctly. If you flex too far forward or extend too far back, it is almost impossible to hit the ball correctly. The only way that you can achieve the correct spine angle and maintain it through the rigors of a golf swing is to have a strong core. Your spine and its motion segments rely on the muscles surrounding them, as well as those in the pelvis, to stabilize them and disperse the forces and loads that occur during the intricate golf swing.

Owing to the fact that the swing is so complicated and the spine angle is so important, an experienced professional golfer who has excellent swing mechanics and is physically fit can still have lower back pain. Not surprisingly, amateur golfers and weekend warriors, who are more likely to have poor swing mechanics, to lack fitness and to avoid proper warm-ups and stretches, are more likely to injure themselves and have chronic, nagging lower back pain.

The lumbar spine is designed to endure stresses that come with everyday motions, such as bending, flexing and rotation. When these stresses are magnified by certain activities, such as a golf swing or a tennis shot, especially when combined with poor technique and poor muscle strength, you overload your spine.

Lessening the Risk of Lower Back Pain When You Play Golf

❶ As with running, you can effectively stabilize and support your spine when you play golf, and overcome the trauma to it by the golf swing, by increasing your core strength and stability. Do the stretches and core exercises in Chapters 2 and 3, as well as in this chapter. The specific exercises on pp. 220–231 will help you with your rotation and the pivot of your pelvis, so that you avoid back pain and improve your swing and ability to hit the golf ball.

❷ Make sure that you have good golf shoes, especially if you are walking the course. They should fit properly, should not be worn down at the heel and should have good arch support, as this will help decrease the stresses to your lumbar spine.

❸ Always warm up properly. Once you're warmed up, practice swinging before playing.

❹ Make sure you breathe properly.

❺ Take lessons, and be sure to ask the pro to show you proper alignment. If the pro doesn't seem to understand spine angle, find one who does!

6 Use a caddy pull-cart if you can't carry a golf bag with dual straps. Always use a golf bag that has a stand so you don't have to bend over to get the clubs.

7 Use the proper lifting technique when picking up the ball, tee and clubs.

8 Walk as much as you can, and stretch as much as you can. As much fun as golf is, playing a few rounds can make for a very long day!

9 Watch the professionals, and pay attention to their stance and their swing.

10 Stretch before and after you play, but if time is short, then stretch afterward.

11 Try using a three-wheeled pushcart, and push it, rather than pulling it, since there is no twisting involved with the pushing motion.

Why Does Golf Cause So Much Back Pain?

There are many culprits:

1. Not stretching prior to practicing or playing a round, and not stretching afterward
2. Poor posture, so you are automatically out of alignment when playing
3. Poor physical condition, especially weak core muscles
4. Not understanding the correct spine angle when swinging
5. Twisting when swinging at the ball
6. Hitting the ground during your swing
7. Hitting balls from awkward locations
8. Bending over to pick up the ball, the tee and the golf clubs
9. Using the wrong equipment based on individual needs (such as your putter's length)
10. Carrying a heavy golf bag or pulling the golf cart, especially over an uneven course
11. Sitting in the golf cart, getting in and out of it, and driving over bumpy terrain

Common Mistakes That Aggravate Your Lower Back When You're Exercising

As a professional, certified trainer, Cara spends a lot of time supervising her clients. She often sees them do things wrong while exercising—things that could cause or exacerbate lower back pain. Back Mindfulness is a must, no matter what kind of exercise you're doing. Always think of your back and how you are using it. Here is a list of common mistakes many people make when exercising:

1. **Improper form.** No matter what exercise or sport you're doing, you need to know how to do it properly—and this is particularly true of working with weights. Ask a certified trainer or coach for advice. Learning how to exercise well is like learning how to do any other activity—it takes a lot of practice. Mastering a sport or an exercise, however, will come much more quickly if your form is good.

2. **Bad posture.** When you slouch or lean forward when you exercise, you put yourself at risk for lower back pain and exacerbate the poor posture you likely have when you aren't exercising.

3. **Leaning over.** Be sure to avoid leaning over while working on cardio machines in the gym, for example. Not only are you putting stress on your spine, shoulders and hips, but you are reducing the effectiveness of your workout if your arms do the work that your legs and core are meant to do because you are tired. Holding on to the handles too tightly can also cause strain; this usually causes you to tense up, which, as you know by now, is not good for your back.

4. **Not concentrating.** It's very easy to zone out while you're exercising, especially while listening to music. This can be great for your relaxation level, but it's dangerous if you're on moving equipment or playing a sport outside. Feel free to listen to music, but just be conscious of your surroundings, too.

5. **Copying others.** It might be tempting to do what a particularly fit exerciser is doing, but your body and skill level might not be similar or a particular routine might not have what your back

needs. Be sure to do what's right for you, not what the person on the treadmill next to you is doing.

6. **Not warming up.** Even when your schedule is frantic and your exercise time is short, always warm up before starting any exercise or weight training.

7. **Not stretching.** Always stretch after your workout.

Don't get discouraged. It can be hard to find the time or the energy to exercise at first, but the more you stick to it, the more you will see results. The rewards are plentiful! If you are new to exercise or have been experiencing pain after working out, hire an experienced trainer who understands lower back pain and can work with you on improving your core strength. If any pain persists, of course, you should seek expert medical advice. Do not self-diagnose!

Beware the Weekend Warrior

Does this sound familiar? You don't exercise or even stretch your muscles all week due to your schedule, so when the weekend comes, you cram in as many physical activities as possible. Perhaps you'll play tennis on Saturday morning, followed by a spinning class at the local gym. On Sunday you'll head out for the afternoon of golf you've been looking forward to all week. Or you'll hit the gym, do a lot of cardio and then lift weights.

Do you stretch before or after any of these activities?

Weekend warriors, who work out only once or twice a week—and often two days in a row—put themselves at risk for lower back pain, especially if they don't stretch. Of course, all forms of exercise are great for your body, mind and spirit—but not if they hurt you because you're trying to cram in too much in too short a time. Exercise doesn't just mean cardio and sweating—it comes in all shapes and forms. Here are some tips for all weekend warriors:

1. Try to get at least thirty minutes of moderate exercise daily. If you can't do it all at once, spread it out, doing fifteen minutes here, fifteen minutes there, and before you know it, you will have

exercised for at least thirty minutes. For example, you already know you need to get up from your desk every so often so your back doesn't bother you, so use this time wisely and pick up the free weights that have been stored under your desk and do some exercises. You can also stretch, as described on pp.146-150 in Chapter 6.

2. Plan ahead, so you don't waste time figuring out what to do.

3. If you know you're going to get home too late to exercise, try to do it on your lunch hour. Exercise for part of your lunch break and eat during the rest.

4. Walk as much as you can: to the train, to your car, up and down stairs, in parking lots. Try carrying light free weights while you're doing a power walk.

Can You Exercise When You Have Back Pain?

As you know already, pain in your lower back is a signal that something has happened. Your body it telling you to stop doing whatever is causing the pain—and stop really does mean stop!

Yet I have seen countless patients over the years who thought they could push past the pain when exercising, and they then unwittingly turned a small, easily correctible situation into something more painful and harder to heal. Of course, I do understand why it is hard to stop exercising; it can be extremely satisfying for stress relief, weight loss and your overall health ... to say nothing of just being a lot of fun!

Many of these patients ask me anxiously if they can keep working out or playing their sport when they have lower back pain. I tell them that there is no one answer, as everyone's injury, sport, core strength and stresses (such as the kind of work you do and how much additional stress it places on your back) are unique. Obviously, if you are injured, you *must* allow for at least six to eight weeks of healing, or follow whatever instructions you have been given by your physician. If you have typical lower back pain from a nonserious injury, you should be able to do the stretches in Chapter 2 every day, which will greatly aid in healing.

Once you have been given the go-ahead to start gently working out again, I recommend that you start with a form of cardio exercise that is non-weight bearing, meaning it does not place stress on your joints. Swimming is often ideal for this.

But whatever causes the least amount of stress to your joints is the best thing, and this depends on the individual and how you are feeling. I have patients who are runners who feel pain and compression in their lower back with each step and can't run at all when they're in pain. Others really do not feel pain when running and may be given the go-ahead to run, within reason (no marathons, please!).

STRETCHING AND CORE ROUTINES FOR SPORTS

What is the one thing the most competent and high-performing professional athletes—from ballet dancers to football players to golfers—have in common? They stretch every day.

RUNNING AND RUNNING SPORTS

Add these stretches to the regular stretching routine in Chapter 2, and follow them with the core routine in Chapter 3.

1. Calf Stretch

❶ Stand upright on a raised object or step.

❷ Put the toes of your right foot on the edge of the object or step. Keep your right leg straight.

❸ Let your right heel drop toward the floor.

④ Hold this position for twenty seconds.

⑤ Repeat this on your left leg.

2. Groin Stretch

① Stand with your feet wider than hip-width apart, toes pointed out.

② Slowly squat down until your knees are directly over your ankles.

③ Place your hands on the tops of your inner thighs and slowly push your thighs outward to open up your hips.

④ Hold the stretch for twenty seconds.

3. Neck Stretch

① Stand upright, arms by your sides.

② Inhale, and then, on the exhale, contract your abdominals and slowly tilt your head to your right shoulder, hold for two to three seconds, and then slowly return to the center.

③ Slowly tilt your head to your left shoulder, hold for two to three seconds, and then slowly return to the center.

④ Bring your chin toward your chest and hold for two to three seconds. Then slowly lift your head up, leaning it back slightly so you are looking up, and hold for two to three seconds. Return slowly to the center. All your movements should be very slow and deliberate.

4. Shoulder Stretch

1 Stand upright, inhale, and then, on the exhale, contract your abdominals.

2 Place your right arm across your chest, and grasp your right elbow with your left hand. Gently pull your right arm across your body.

3 Hold this position for twenty seconds.

4 Repeat with your left arm.

5. Chest Stretch

1 Stand facing a sturdy pole, the edge of a doorway or a wall, and grab hold of it with your right hand.

2 Contract your abdominals, and then slowly pivot your feet and rotate your body to your left, away from the pole, doorway or wall (which will now be behind you). You should feel the stretch in your chest, just above your right breast.

3 Hold the abdominal contraction for fifteen seconds, and then switch to your left side. Remember to keep breathing evenly.

RACQUET SPORTS

Add these exercises to your core routine.

For the next two exercises, pick the one that is most comfortable for you to do.

1a. Push-up on Knees

1 Kneel on the floor, with your arms straight and aligned so that your hands are shoulder-width apart facing forward or are turned in slightly, and with your feet off the floor.

2 Inhale, and then, on the exhale, contract your abdominals.

3 Inhale, bending your elbows, lower your body until your chest gets close to the floor, pause, exhale and push back up to the starting position. Make sure you don't arch your back or let it sag, and keep your neck aligned with your spine. Look down, not up.

4 Do this ten times.

1b. Push-up with Straight Legs

1 Kneel on the floor, with your arms straight and aligned so that your hands are shoulder-width apart facing forward or are turned in slightly.

2 Inhale, and then, on the exhale, contract your abdominals and extend your legs behind you.

3 Inhale, bending your elbows, lower your body until your chest gets close to the floor, pause, exhale and push back up to the starting position. Make sure you don't arch your back or let it sag, and keep your neck aligned with your spine. Look down, not up.

4 Do this ten times.

For the next two exercises, pick the one that is most comfortable for you to do.

2a. Kneel Twist with Racquet or Towel

1 Holding a racquet or a towel, kneel down with your right knee in front of you, your right foot flat on the mat, your left knee on the mat behind you and your left foot facing down. You can place a pillow under your knee for comfort.

2 Inhale, and then, on the exhale, contract your abdominals and twist the racquet or towel toward your right side, then back to your center. Make sure you twist just past your shoulder.

3 Repeat on your left side.

4 Do this ten times.

2b. Lunge Twist with Racquet or Towel

1 Stand upright with a racquet or towel in your hands.

2 Inhale, and then, on the exhale, contract your abdominals and lunge forward with your right leg. Your right leg should be in a bent-knee position, and your left leg should be behind you, with your heel raised.

3 Twist the racquet or towel toward your right side, just past your right shoulder, then back to your center.

4 Repeat on your left side.

5 Do this ten to twenty times.

For the next three exercises, pick the one that is most comfortable for you to do.

3a. Lying Side-to-Side Rotation

1 Lie on your back, knees bent, arms at your sides on the floor.

2 Inhale, and then, on the exhale, contract your abdominals and bring your right knee and then your left knee up to chest height.

3 Bring your arms up to your sides, creating a T formation with your body.

4 With abdominals contracted, slowly bring both knees to your right side, making sure your head, shoulders and arms remain on the mat, and then slowly bring your knees to the left side. This is a small movement, so don't go too far over to each side. Keep your abdominals contracted during the entire exercise.

5 Lower your knees one at a time.

6 Do this ten times.

3b. Lying Side-to-Side Rotation with Stability Ball

1 Lie on your back, knees bent, holding a stability ball in your hands.

2 Inhale, and then, on the exhale, contract your abdominals, straighten your legs and place the ball between your feet, or keep your knees bent with the ball between them.

3 Place your arms out at your sides in a T formation.

4 With your abdominals contracted, slowly bring your legs with the ball to your right side, making sure your head, shoulders and arms remain on the mat, and then slowly bring your legs to your left side. Don't go too far over to each side; just go past your shoulders.

5 Do this ten times.

4. Calf Stretch

1 Stand with something sturdy in front of you to hold on to, feet facing forward, shoulder-width apart.

2 Inhale, and then, on the exhale, contract your abdominals, rise up on to your toes, and then slowly lower yourself down to the starting position.

3 Do this ten times.

STRETCHES BEFORE YOU PLAY

Do the seven stretches now. When you are done, add on the following stretches.

1. Neck Stretch

1 Stand upright, arms by your sides.

2 Inhale, and then, on the exhale, contract your abdominals and slowly tilt your head to your right shoulder, hold for two to three seconds, and then slowly return to the center.

3 Slowly tilt your head to your left shoulder, and hold for two to three seconds, and then slowly return to the center.

4 Bring your chin toward your chest and hold for two to three seconds. Then slowly lift your head up, leaning it back slightly so you are looking up, and hold for two to three seconds. Return slowly to the center. All your movements should be very slow and deliberate.

2. Shoulder Stretch

1 Stand upright, inhale, and then, on the exhale, contract your abdominals.

2 Place your right arm across your chest, and grasp your right elbow with your left hand. Gently pull your right arm across your body.

3 Hold this position for twenty seconds.

4 Repeat with your left arm.

3. Chest Stretch

1 Stand facing a sturdy pole, the edge of a doorway or a wall, and grab hold of it with your right hand.

2 Contract your abdominals, and then slowly pivot your feet and rotate your body to your left, away from the pole, doorway or wall (which will now be behind you). You should feel the stretch in your chest, just above your right breast.

3 Hold the stretch for twenty seconds, and then switch to your left side. Remember to keep breathing evenly.

4. Tricep Stretch with Towel

1 Hold a towel in your left hand. Stand upright, inhale, and then, on the exhale, contract your abdominals.

2 Lift the towel over your left shoulder, and then use your right hand to reach behind your back and pull the other end of the towel down.

3 Hold the stretch for twenty seconds.

4 Repeat on the right side.

On the Court

Court Stretches

If your back gets tight while playing, you can do these seated stretches from a bench or chair and the standing ones as well.

1. Standing Hamstring Stretch

1 Stand upright, facing a bench.

2 Inhale, and then, on the exhale, contract your abdominals and place your right heel on the bench.

3 Place your right hand on your right leg and your left hand on your left leg.

4 Slightly bend your left knee, and slowly lower your upper body down toward your right leg.

5 Hold the stretch for thirty seconds.

6 Slowly raise your upper body until you are upright, and repeat with your left leg.

7 You can do this two times with each leg if your muscles are tight.

2. Seated Spinal Twist

1 Sit tall with your feet flat on the floor, hip-width apart, your back touching the back of the seat, and your arms at your sides.

2 Inhale, and then, on the exhale, contract your abdominals.

3 Cross your left leg over your right leg, place your right hand on the side of your left knee, and then turn your body to the left while your left hand and arm go behind you. You should be looking to your left. Hold for ten to twenty seconds.

4 Then cross your right leg over your left leg, place your left hand on the side of your right knee, and then turn your body to the right while your right hand and arm go behind you. You should be looking to your right. Hold for ten to twenty seconds.

3. Seated Piriformis Stretch

1 Sit tall on a chair with your feet flat on the floor, hip-width apart, your back touching the back of the seat.

2 Inhale, and then, on the exhale, contract your abdominals.

3 Cross your right leg over your left leg so that your right ankle is resting on your left thigh.

4 Place your left hand on your right ankle and your right hand on your right knee, and then slowly lower your upper body down toward them. Stop lowering yourself as soon as you feel the stretch in the right piriformis muscle, located on the side of your right hip and buttock. Do not round your back.

5 Hold this position for fifteen seconds, and then switch, this time crossing your left leg over your right leg.

4. Quadriceps Standing Stretch

1 Stand next to something sturdy, and hold on to it with your left hand.

2 Grasp your right foot (or ankle, if that's easier) with your right hand, and gently pull your leg back and up, with your toes pointing toward your head. Make sure your left knee remains straight.

3 Hold this position for thirty seconds.

4 Switch to your left leg and repeat.

5. Total Back Stretch

1 Stand with something sturdy in front of you, and bend your knees. Contract your abdominals, and then grasp the object with both hands, keeping your arms straight. Keep your head level with your shoulders.

2 Hold this position for ten to twenty seconds.

3 Stand up straight, place your right hand on your waist and your left arm up over your head, and then side bend to the right.

4 Hold this position for ten seconds, and then switch sides.

6. Shoulder Stretch

1 Stand upright, inhale, and then, on the exhale, contract your abdominals.

2 Place your right arm across your chest, and grasp your right elbow with your left hand. Gently pull your right arm across your body.

❸ Hold this position for twenty seconds.

❹ Repeat with your left arm.

7. Chest Stretch

❶ Stand facing a sturdy object, and grab hold of it with your right hand.

❷ Contract your abdominals, and then slowly pivot your feet and rotate your body to your left, away from the object (which will now be behind you). You should feel the stretch in your chest, just above your right breast.

❸ Hold the stretch for fifteen seconds, and then switch to your left side. Remember to keep breathing evenly.

8. Tricep Stretch with Towel

❶ Hold a towel in your left hand. Stand upright, inhale, and then, on the exhale, contract your abdominals.

❷ Lift the towel over your left shoulder, and then use your right hand to reach behind your back and pull the other end of the towel down.

❸ Hold the stretch for twenty seconds.

❹ Repeat on the right side.

GOLF

This routine should be done in addition to the core routine in Chapter 3. Start slow and go at your own pace. Remember to always warm up before you start, and do the seven stretches when you are finished with the core routine. Do only the core routine in Chapter 3 on the days you are not playing golf.

The next two exercises are not meant to be done in the same session. Pick the one that is most comfortable for you to do.

1a. Push-up on Knees

1 Kneel on the floor, with your arms straight and aligned so that your hands are shoulder-width apart facing forward or are turned in slightly, and with your feet off the floor.

2 Inhale, and then, on the exhale, contract your abdominals and do a slight Pelvic Tilt to place yourself in the correct position.

3 Inhale, bending your elbows, lower your body until your chest gets close to the floor, pause, exhale and push back up to the starting position. Make sure you don't arch your back or let it sag, and keep your neck aligned with your spine. Look down, not up.

4 Do this ten times.

1b. Push-up with Straight Legs

1 Kneel on the floor, with your arms straight and aligned so that your hands are shoulder-width apart facing forward or are turned in slightly.

② Inhale, and then, on the exhale, contract your abdominals, do a slight Pelvic Tilt to place yourself in the correct position, and extend your legs behind you. Your weight should be on your toes.

③ Inhale, bending your elbows, lower your body until your chest gets close to the floor, pause, exhale and push back up to the starting position. Make sure you don't arch your back or let it sag, and keep your neck aligned with your spine. Look down, not up.

④ Do this ten times.

The next two exercises are not meant to be done in the same session. Pick the one that is most comfortable for you to do.

2a. Kneel Twist with Golf Club or Towel

① While holding a golf club or a towel, kneel down with your right knee in front of you, your right foot flat on the mat, your left knee on the mat behind you and your left foot facing down. You can place a pillow under your knee for comfort.

② Inhale, and then, on the exhale, contract your abdominals and twist the golf club or towel toward your right side, then back to your center. Make sure you twist just past your shoulder.

③ Repeat on your left side.

④ Do this ten times.

2b. Lunge Twist with Golf Club or Towel

1 Stand upright with a golf club or towel in your hands.

2 Inhale, and then, on the exhale, contract your abdominals and lunge forward with your right leg. Your right leg should be in a bent-knee position, and your left leg should be behind you, with your heel raised.

3 Twist the golf club or towel toward your right side, just past your right shoulder, then back to your center.

4 Repeat on your left side.

5 Do this ten to twenty times.

3a. Lying Side-to-Side Rotation

1 Lie on your back, knees bent, arms at your sides on the floor.

2 Inhale, and then, on the exhale, contract your abdominals and bring your right knee and then your left knee up to chest height.

3 Bring your arms up to your sides, creating a T formation with your body.

4 With abdominals contracted, slowly bring both knees to your right side, making sure your head, shoulders and arms remain on the mat, and then slowly bring your knees to the left side. This is a small movement, so don't go too far over to each side. Keep your abdominals contracted during the entire exercise.

5 Lower your knees one at a time.

6 Do this ten times.

3b. Lying Side-to-Side Rotation with Stability Ball

1 Lie on your back, knees bent, holding a stability ball in your hands.

2 Inhale, and then, on the exhale, contract your abdominals, straighten your legs and place the ball between your feet, or keep your knees bent with the ball between them.

3 Place your arms out at your sides in a T formation.

4 With your abdominals contracted, slowly bring your legs with the ball to your right side, making sure your head, shoulders and arms remain on the mat, and then slowly bring your legs to your left side. Don't go too far over to each side; just go past your shoulders.

5 Do this ten times.

4. Calf Stretch

1 Stand with something sturdy in front of you to hold on to, feet facing forward, shoulder-width apart.

2 Inhale, and then, on the exhale, contract your abdominals, rise up on to your toes, and then slowly lower yourself down to the starting position.

3 Do this ten times.

5. Back Row with Band

1 Place an exercise band around a sturdy object at torso level. Stand with your knees bent, facing the object, and hold the band with two hands, palms facing in.

2 Inhale, and then, on the exhale, contract your abdominals.

3 Pull the band back toward your body so that your hands are near your chest, keeping your elbows close to your body.

4 As you pull back, squeeze your shoulder blades together, and then slowly release the band and go back to the starting position.

5 Repeat with your palms facing down.

6 Repeat with your palms facing up.

7 Do this ten times.

Stretches Before You Play

Do the seven stretches now. When you are done, add on the following stretches.

1. Neck Stretch

1 Stand upright, arms by your sides.

2 Inhale, and then, on the exhale, contract your abdominals and slowly tilt your head to your right shoulder, hold for two to three seconds, and then slowly return to the center.

3 Slowly tilt your head to your left shoulder, hold for two to three seconds, and then slowly return to the center.

4 Bring your chin toward your chest, hold for two to three seconds. Then slowly lift your head up, leaning it back slightly so you are looking up, and hold for two to three seconds. Return slowly to the center. All your movements should be very slow and deliberate.

2. Shoulder Stretch

1 Stand upright, inhale, and then, on the exhale, contract your abdominals.

2 Place your right arm across your chest, and grasp your right elbow with your left hand. Gently pull your right arm across your body.

3 Hold this position for twenty seconds.

4 Repeat with your left arm.

3. Chest Stretch

1 Stand facing a sturdy pole, the edge of a doorway or a wall, and grab hold of it with your right hand.

2 Contract your abdominals, slowly pivot your feet and rotate your body to your left, away from the pole, doorway or wall (which will now be behind you). You should feel the stretch in your chest, just above your right breast.

3 Hold the stretch for fifteen seconds, then switch to your left side. Remember to keep breathing evenly.

4. Tricep Stretch with Golf Club or Towel

1 Hold a lightweight golf club or towel in your left hand. Stand upright, inhale, and then, on the exhale, contract your abdominals.

2 Lift the golf club or towel over your left shoulder, and then use your right hand to reach behind your back and pull the other end of the golf club or towel down.

3 Hold the stretch for twenty seconds.

4 Repeat on the right side.

On the Golf Course

Pre-swing Stretch

This stretches you and warms you up to play.

1. Towel or Golf Club Swing

1 Stand in your golf stance, holding a towel or golf club in front of you.

2 Inhale, and then, on the exhale, contract your abdominals.

3 Swing the towel or golf club diagonally up to the right and then to the left. Do not move your lower body.

4 Do this ten to twenty times.

Golf Course Stretches

If your back gets tight while playing, you can do these seated stretches from the golf cart and the standing ones as well.

1. Standing Hamstring Stretch

1 Stand upright, facing the golf cart.

2 Inhale, and then, on the exhale, contract your abdominals and place your right heel on the floor of the golf cart.

3 Place your right hand on your right leg and your left hand on your left leg. If you need more support, hold on to the cart itself.

4 Slightly bend your left knee, and slowly lower your upper body down toward your right leg.

5 Hold the stretch for thirty seconds.

6 Slowly raise your upper body until you are upright, and repeat with your left leg.

7 You can do this two times with each leg if your muscles are tight.

Do the next two exercises only if you have enough room.

2. Seated Spinal Twist

1 Sit tall in the golf cart with your feet flat on the floor, hip-width apart, your back touching the back of the seat.

2 Inhale, and then, on the exhale, contract your abdominals.

3 Cross your left leg over your right leg, place both arms over to your left side, and slowly twist at your waist so you can look over to your right shoulder.

4 Hold for ten to twenty seconds, and then switch to your left side.

3. Seated Piriformis Stretch

1 Sit tall in the golf cart with your feet flat on the floor, hip-width apart, your back touching the back of the seat.

2 Inhale, and then, on the exhale, contract your abdominals.

3 Cross your right leg over your left leg so that your right ankle is resting on your left thigh.

4 Place your left hand on your right ankle and your right hand on your right knee, and then slowly lower your upper body down toward them. Stop lowering yourself as soon as you feel the stretch in the right piriformis muscle, located on the side of your right hip and buttock. Do not round your back.

5 Hold this position for fifteen seconds, and then switch, this time crossing your left leg over your right leg.

4. Quadriceps Standing Stretch

1 Stand next to the golf cart, and hold on to it with your left hand.

2 Grasp your right foot (or ankle, if that's easier) with your right hand, and gently pull your leg back and up, with your toes pointing toward your head. Make sure your left knee remains straight.

3 Hold this position for thirty seconds.

4 Switch to your left leg and repeat.

5. Total Back Stretch

1 Stand with the golf cart in front of you, and bend your knees. Contract your abdominals, and then grasp the golf cart with both hands, keeping your arms straight. Keep your head level with your shoulders.

2 Hold this position for ten to twenty seconds.

3 Stand up straight, place your right hand on your waist and your left arm up over your head, and then bend to the right.

4 Hold this position for ten seconds, and then switch sides.

6. Chest Stretch

1 Stand facing the golf cart, and grab hold of it with your right hand.

2 Contract your abdominals, slowly pivot your feet and rotate your body to your left, away from the cart (which will now be behind you). You should feel the stretch in your chest, just above your right breast.

3 Hold the stretch for fifteen seconds, and then switch to your left side. Remember to keep breathing evenly.

4 If you don't have a golf cart, use a sturdy object, like a tree.

7. Triceps Stretch with Golf Club or Towel

1 Hold a lightweight golf club or towel in your left hand. Stand upright, inhale, and then, on the exhale, contract your abdominals.

2 Lift the golf club or towel over your left shoulder, and then use your right hand to reach behind your back and pull the other end of the golf club or towel down.

3 Hold this position for twenty seconds.

4 Repeat on the right side.

8. Forearm Stretch Fingers Down

1 Stand upright, inhale, and then, on the exhale, contract your abdominals.

2 With your right arm straight out in front of you, turn it so your palm is facing away from you, fingers facing down.

3 With your left hand, press your right fingers toward you.

4 Hold the stretch for ten to twenty seconds.

5 Repeat on the left hand.

The Best Alignment for Golf

1. Your feet, hips, forearms, shoulders and eyes should be parallel to the target line.

2. Your feet should be shoulder-width apart.

3. Keep your weight on the insteps of your feet, with your knees slightly flexed over them.

4. Find your ideal spine angle before swinging.

5. Bend at your hips, not your waist, with your buttocks slightly sticking out.

6. Try not to put any stress on your quadriceps (front of your thighs).

7. Contract your abdominal muscles when bending, lifting and riding in the golf cart.

IF YOU DO NEED MEDICAL TREATMENT FOR YOUR LOWER BACK PAIN

WHEN MY PATIENTS FIRST COME TO ME, almost all of them are convinced that the severity of their pain automatically means they will need back surgery. I tell them that only about 40 percent of lower back pain sufferers will actually need more intensive treatment, and of that number, even fewer will need surgery.

Every patient is different, of course, and treatment must be tailored to each case, but these are the most common noninvasive procedures that are prescribed first.

NONINVASIVE PROCEDURES FOR LOWER BACK PAIN

My patients who need more intense treatment for lower back pain or other back pain are usually prescribed a series of treatments, consisting of some or all of the following:

- The seven stretches and core-strengthening exercises. These can be done by all patients.

- Physical therapy. This might include ultrasound, heat or cold packs, targeted exercises, massage therapy and transcutaneous electrical nerve stimulation (TENS, a painless electrical current that pinpoints specific nerves).

- Chiropractic care.

- Injections of steroids. Steroids are used in conjunction with the preceding treatments for those patients who have not improved with physical therapy or who have sciatica.

The overwhelming majority of my lower back pain patients recover after these treatments. If, however, there is no relief after these non-operative treatments have been tried, only then would surgical options be explored.

ARE YOU REALLY A CANDIDATE FOR LOWER BACK SURGERY?

Decades ago, surgery for lower back pain and other issues was less scientific and results were less predictable, making patients apprehensive about any procedures. Now, with so many new, minimally invasive and highly successful techniques, surgery is no longer something to fear.

If you do need back surgery, there are two goals: one is to decompress the nerve if it's causing sciatic-like symptoms, and the other is to stabilize or neutralize a motion segment when pain is due to disc degeneration, or from instability or deformity of a motion segment (see pp. 11–13 in Chapter 1).

PROCEDURE	LUMBAR FUSION
What It Does	This procedure fuses the motion segment to alleviate pain and stop the painful motion of this part of the spine. It can be performed both open or minimally invasive, depending on the specific problem.
Procedure Length	2-3 hours, depending on how many levels need to be fused.

Recuperation Time	6 weeks. Patients can usually start physical therapy as early as 3 weeks post-procedure and can get aggressive with early activity to rejuvenate their back muscles.
Pain Factor	Moderate for only a few days to a week, and then minimal as the patient becomes more mobile.
Expected Results	Relief of pain and return to normal activity level.
Will This Take Care of the Problem for Good?	Yes, at the segment that is fused.

PROCEDURE	DISCECTOMY
What It Does	This is a microsurgical procedure to remove a herniated, or "ruptured," disc that has been causing sciatica.
Procedure Length	½ hour.
Recuperation Time	Minimal.
Pain Factor	Minimal incisional pain, and relief of sciatica almost immediately post-surgery.
Expected Results	98 percent successful.
Will This Take Care of the Problem for Good?	Yes.

HOW TO FIND A QUALIFIED ORTHOPEDIC SURGEON IN YOUR AREA

A well-informed patient is one who is proactive before and after surgery. Being well-informed starts with finding the best surgeon for your needs. I have been a contributor and editor at www.spineuniverse.com

for over ten years, and it is an extremely helpful source for finding a physician or surgeon and educating yourself about back problems and surgical options.

Try to cover the topics discussed below with the office staff prior to your consultation, so you can spend as much time as possible with your physician or surgeon talking about your pain or other issues. Once you have covered these topics prior to your appointment, be sure to write down any questions and take them with you, as it is easy to forget what you want to ask during your appointment! Here are the topics:

Board Certification

It is very important that patients do due diligence and ask about the board certification of their surgeon of choice. Valid board certification indicates that the person has completed training, passed rigorous examinations and continued to update their knowledge annually. In orthopedics we have to renew our board certification every ten years. In most states, insurance companies require surgeons to be board certified in order to participate. Orthopedic surgeons should be certified by the American Board of Orthopaedic Surgery; neurosurgeons, who often perform back surgery, should be certified by the American Association of Neurological Surgeons. (There is no specific certification for a "spine surgeon" as that is a subspecialty of orthopedic surgery.) Following residency, physicians and surgeons do a fellowship for one year in their field of interest. In my case it was a spine fellowship. I would recommend that if you need spine surgery, you seek out a surgeon who has been fellowship trained.

For more details, see http://www.spineuniverse.com/treatments/ surgery/neurosurgeon-or-orthopedic-surgeon-does-matter.

Membership Organizations

Spine surgeons also keep up to date with the latest techniques and procedures through membership in peer organizations. I am a member of the North American Spine Society, the American Academy of Orthopaedic Surgeons and the American Society of Spine Surgeons. Most surgeons find these organizations critical to maintaining knowledge in their specialty.

Hospital Affiliation

You need to know where your spine surgeon has attending privileges and is permitted to perform surgery. Is this location convenient for you? Is this a highly rated facility?

Years of Experience with This Procedure

Any orthopedic surgeon will have had basic training in spine procedures while doing advanced training in medical school/residency before becoming board certified, but it is in your best interest to work with a spine surgeon with extensive experience doing the particular procedure you need. Many surgeons are brilliant at one or a few specific techniques, because that is their specialty, but they are less skilled at procedures they do infrequently. Ask your surgeon how long he or she has trained in your particular procedure, and how many procedures he or she has already performed.

Peer-Reviewed Publications
about This Procedure

Surgeons who are skilled at certain procedures and techniques, and at the use of new devices, often write about them for peer-reviewed professional publications.

Complaint Registries

The internet has made it easy to research nearly any topic, but it has also encouraged anonymous comment posting, and such comments can often be highly misleading. Be very wary of internet sites that allow people to rate physicians and surgeons, as they are usually biased and inaccurate. The only truly valid sources for complaints are the state licensing board and the professional societies for that physician's or surgeon's specialty.

Rapport

A good surgeon understands your fears and seeks to put you at ease. I love talking to my patients and answering their questions. But if you really don't click with a surgeon's personality, for whatever reason, it really is okay to find a different surgeon—one who makes you feel comfortable. (Confident surgeons will encourage you to get a second opinion so you can make a more informed decision.) You certainly don't want to add any additional stress or worries to the process.

ACKNOWLEDGMENTS

First and foremost, we would like to thank our families for their unwavering support and patience through the creation of this book: Gerard's wife Elise, son Jordan and daughter Sydney; and Cara's husband Allen, son Logan and daughter Sydney.

This book would not have come together without the following people, to whom we are profoundly grateful: Karen Moline, whose insight and knowledge about writing have been invaluable; Deborah Brody and the staff at Harlequin for believing in this book and doing such an amazing job publishing it; and our agent, Stephanie Tade, for her peerless direction and enthusiasm. We would also like to thank Scott Wynn and his team for the photographs and Victoria Skomal Wilchinsky for the illustrations.

We are forever humbled by the millions who suffer from chronic back pain, and hope that we will make a difference in your lives.

INDEX

Page numbers of illustrations appear in italics.